TOTALLY FIT

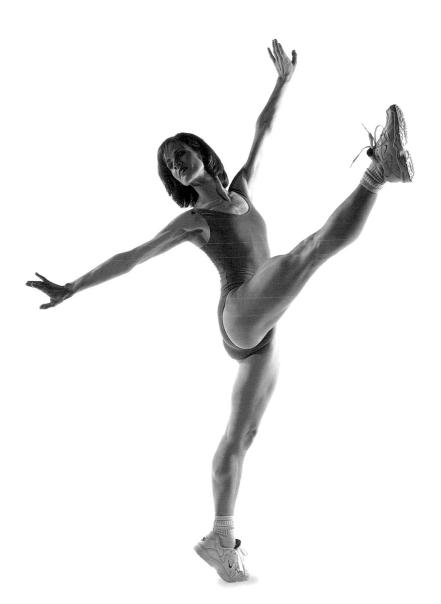

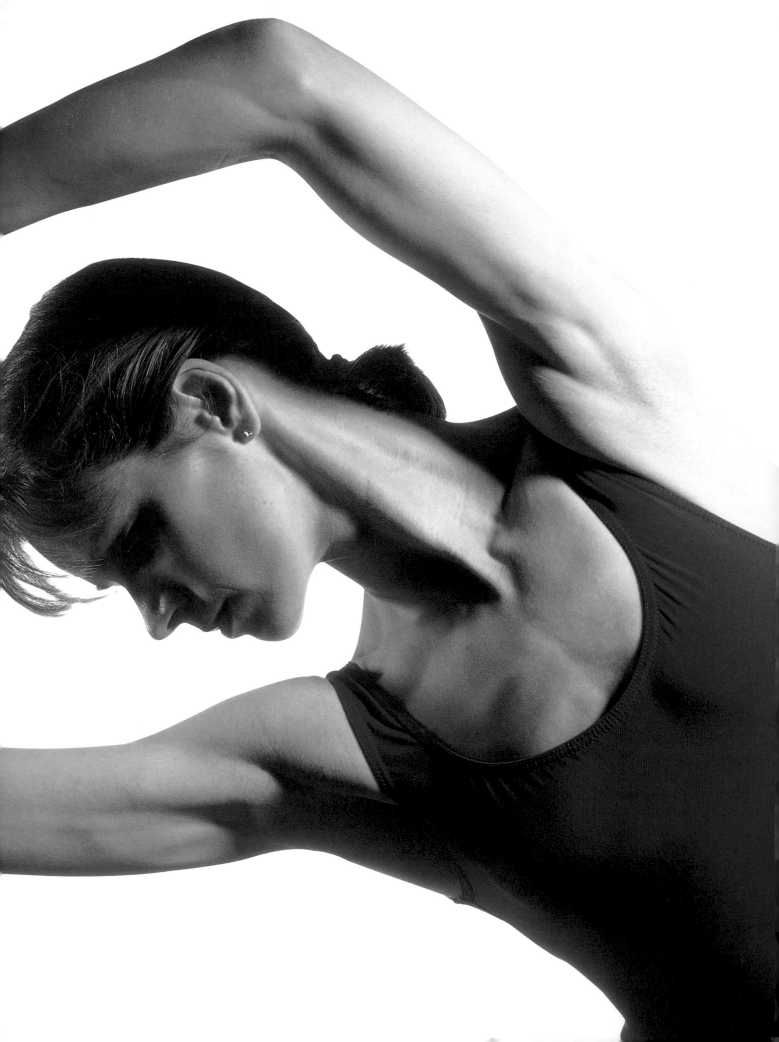

TOTALLY FIT

Deborah Bull

DK PUBLISHING, INC.

DK

A DK PUBLISHING BOOK

Project Editor Monica Chakraverty

Art Editor Robert Ford

Editor David Summers

Designer Claudia Norris

Senior Art Editor Tracey Clarke

DTP Designer Karen Ruane

Managing Editor Susannah Marriott/Mary Ling

Managing Art Editor Toni Kay

Photographers Dave King, Andy Crawford

Production Manager Maryann Rogers

"Nobody gets it wrong on purpose."
(after Socrates)

For Torje, who made sense of it all.

First American Edition, 1998

2 4 6 8 10 9 7 5 3 1

Published in the United States by
DK Publishing, Inc., 95 Madison Avenue New York, New York 10016
Visit us on the World Wide Web at http://www.dk.com

Library of Congress Cataloging-in-Publication Data
Bull, Deborah.
Totally Fit / by Deborah Bull and Torje Eike. – 1st American ed.
p. cm.
Includes index.
ISBN 0-7894-2990-X
1. Weight loss. 2. Physical Fitness. 3. Exercise. I. Eike, Torje. II. Title.
RM222.2.B84 1998   97-38636
613.7--dc21   CIP

Reproduced in Singapore by Colourscan
Printed and bound in England by Butler and Tanner

Contents

FOREWORD 6

FIT FOR LIFE 7

Weight Loss: The Facts 10

*Understanding how the body works and
how to work with it to lose weight*

The Myths 12

The Facts 14

Using Energy 16

Diet or Exercise? 18

What is Exercise? 19

Which Type of Exercise? 20

Reading Your Heart Rate 22

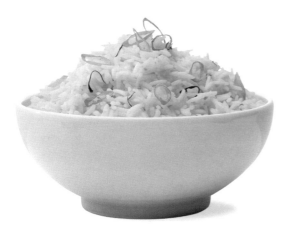

Energy for Life 24

*A complete nutrition guide explains the
fundamentals of a healthy diet*

The Lowdown on Calories 26

Carbohydrates 28

Protein 30

Fat 32

Vitamins & Minerals 34

Water 36

Striking a Balance 38

How to Read Food Labels 40

Seven-point Plan 41

The Good Food Guides 42

The Good Breakfast Guide 43

The Good Lunch Guide 44

The Good Dinner Guide 46

The Good Snack Guide 48

Total Fitness Plan 50

*A fitness package to last a lifetime, with an
effective exercise routine to tone the whole body*

Getting the Right Gear 52

When to Exercise 54

The Pre-Exercise Plan 55

The Fitness Plan 56

Warm Up 57

Light Stretch 58

Aerobic Exercise 60

5-minute Cool-down 63

Strength Training 64

Abdominals 65 ▪ Back Extensions 66

Chair Dips 68 ▪ Hamstrings 70

Biceps 72 ▪ Arabesque 74

Inner Thigh 76 ▪ Deltoid 78

Stretches 80

Inner Thigh 81 ▪ Hip Flexor 82

Front Thigh 84 ▪ Hamstrings 85

Upper Calf 86 ▪ Lower Calf 87

Side Stretch 88 ▪ Cat Stretch 90

Hanging Stretch 91

GLOSSARY 92

INDEX 93–95

ADDRESSES 96

ACKNOWLEDGMENTS 96

Foreword

WHENEVER I WATCH DEBORAH BULL DANCE, I am amazed by how great she looks and how much energy she seems to have. *Totally Fit* tells you just how she does it. In this book, she gives you the information you need to help you maximize your energy yet still control your weight.

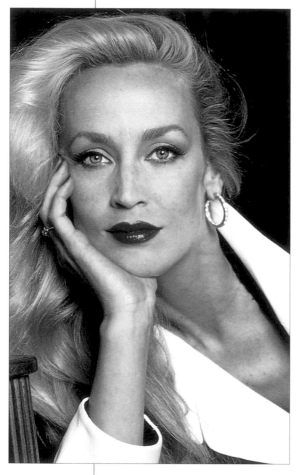

In all the years I've been modeling, I've come across many weird and wonderful diets. Yet in the long run, none of them ever work, because, as Deborah says, losing weight is not about the things you should not do, it's about the things you should do. There is no need to starve yourself in order to stay slim, and you don't need expensive gyms or exercise equipment to stay fit. Like me, Deborah follows Torje Eike's Total Fitness Plan, a routine I have used for years to keep myself in shape. If you are fed up with dieting but want to stay in shape, I can't think of two better people to tell you how.

JERRY HALL

Fit for Life

ACCORDING TO THE LATEST RESEARCH, one in six of us is obese; in the United States, this figure is as high as one in three. It is, therefore, hardly surprising that we are obsessed with diet. For some of us, getting thin has become an all-consuming passion, and there is apparently no limit to what we will not swallow in the hope of losing weight. Even when it seems that the market must have reached the saturation point, another "miracle diet" tops the bestseller list.

The Secret of Permanent Weight Loss

The sad truth, however, is that where diets are concerned, there are no miracles. If there were, the problem of obesity would have been solved long ago and this book would not exist. Let's be quite clear from the start: if a diet makes you eat less, it will also make you lose weight. Unfortunately, you won't lose it *permanently*. As soon as you come off the diet and begin to eat normally again, your weight will creep upward and, before long, you will be back where you started.

You just cannot lose weight fast *and* lose it permanently, and a diet book that promises a slimmer figure in days should carry a subtitle guaranteeing the old one back in a matter of weeks. If this were just another of those books, you could stop reading now. But it isn't. This book does not just tell you how to lose weight: it tells you how to put weight problems behind you forever, so that you can get on with enjoying life.

The Dancer's Diet

The idea of taking advice on diet from a ballet dancer might seem a little strange. After all, aren't all dancers naturally blessed with perfect bodies? Surely they know nothing about struggling to control their weight. But think about it a little longer: your idea of a ballet dancer is probably two-sided. On the one hand is an image of a waiflike creature who weighs less than her pointe shoes. On the other are the horror stories about the lengths to which dancers will go to reach that state of perfection.

Dancers, who in reality are of the same flesh and blood as everyone else, are usually fighting exactly the same battle with their bodies. Until recently, I was no exception. Like many dancers, I have in the past had a rather "special" relationship with food. For the first twelve years of my professional life, I was in constant conflict with my body, struggling to maintain the sylphlike silhouette of a ballerina while still having enough energy to get up and dance. The two requirements did not seem compatible: I was born with the classic "pear" shape – hips wider than shoulders – and what seemed like an unconquerable tendency to gain weight. I tried every trick in the book (and some which are not) to combat weight gain, in an endless cycle of yo-yo dieting with low-calorie, one-meal-a-day, near-starvation, and salad-and-fruit-only diets. Some diets were more successful than others and the weight would drop off, but the end result was always the same and, within a week or so, the weight was back on again. By cutting down on the calories in my diet, I assumed I was cutting down on the fat, but managed instead to cut the energy I so vitally needed to dance.

Vital Statistics

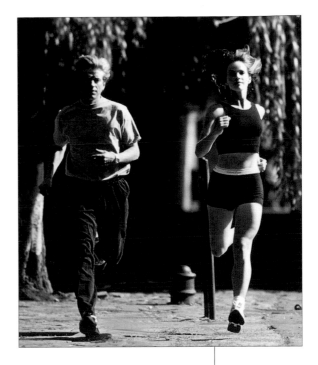

I had almost given up the fight when I met Torje Eike in 1993. With his expert knowledge of the way the body works, he introduced me to a concept of eating based on physiology: fact rather than fiction. All my previous convictions about diet were turned on their heads. For a long time I had avoided bread, pasta, and other forms of carbohydrates, in the belief that they were fattening, but Torje insisted that they were precisely the foods I should be eating – they were the source of the energy I so badly needed. It was this connection between food and fuel that started me on a journey of discovery. I gave up the search for a magic formula for weight loss, and finally found what I was looking for in the physiology of the human body itself.

Losing and controlling weight became no more than a question of accepting that the body runs better on some fuels than others. If, like me, you thought dieting was about self-deprivation, starvation, and agonizing sessions in the gym, you're in for a very pleasant surprise: losing weight is not about the things you should not do – it is about the things you *should* do.

DEBORAH BULL

Weight Loss : The Facts

No matter how many failed diets we have under our belts, it is still tempting to believe that somewhere there is a miracle diet that will help us lose pounds without any effort at all. I spent years searching for it and was taken in, time and time again, by the fresh and seductive promise of a magic formula for weight loss.

Yet, however many diets I tried, I never managed to lose weight permanently. It was only when I started to work with my body – rather than fight against it – that my personal battle became a thing of the past. It is the facts that provide the answers, and you need to understand those facts before weight control makes sense. It may all seem a little complicated at first, but persevere: battling with a few pages of information is going to be a lot easier than battling against your body.

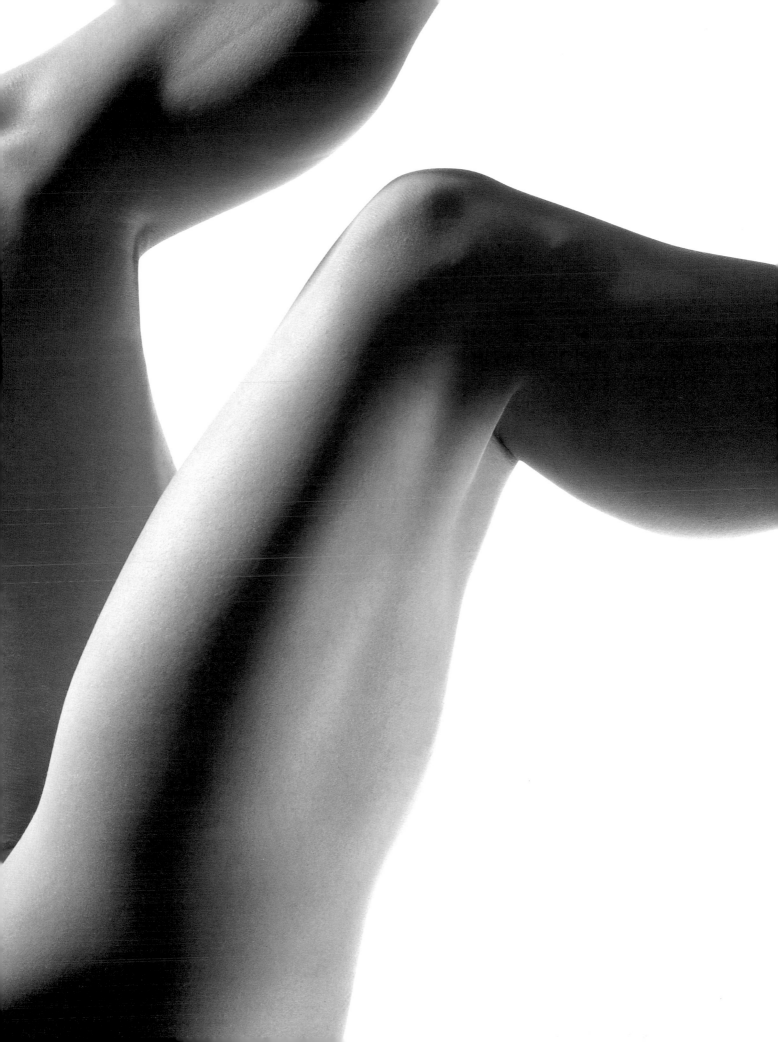

The Myths

The human body is like a machine; it operates according to certain laws that cannot be ignored. Until I understood those laws, I tried every possible way to get thin, but failed with remarkable consistency: I had the will to succeed but lacked the knowledge. But before we face the facts, let's dispel a few myths.

1 The only way to lose weight is to eat less

It is unquestionably true that you can lose "weight" by eating less. Everyone has done it at some point, either through choice or illness. Depriving your body of the food it needs can undoubtedly lead to rapid loss of body mass. Whether it leads to rapid loss of *fat* is another matter. It is unlikely that there is any way, apart from surgery, that fat can be lost rapidly. Furthermore, scientific research proves that weight loss through diet alone is successful in the long term less than 20% of the time, and in some studies it's even less.

2 The scales never lie

Unfortunately they do. Rapid weight loss looks so good on the scales because it is mainly a loss of water and muscle. Muscle, being compact, weighs much more than fat, so two people can weigh the same yet look very different. The best way to assess progress is to:
■ Throw away your scales.
■ Dig out an old pair of jeans that fit when you were happy with your body. Try them on at regular intervals until you can fasten the zipper.
■ Congratulate yourself and keep going.

3 If I eat less than I need, my body will need to burn its excess fat

This would seem to be logical. We all have a lot of fat stored up and it is, in some circumstances, a very efficient source of energy. Unfortunately it's not in this circumstance. Your body's first priority is always to protect the brain. The brain depends on glucose, from carbohydrates, for its fuel. Fat cannot be converted into glucose but, in emergencies – when no carbohydrates are eaten – protein can. When starved, the body turns to its protein stores to provide energy, and you start to "eat" your own muscles.

4 Certain exercises burn fat from specific areas

The theory behind "spot reducing" is that muscle activity in a specific area stimulates the burning of the fat deposits closest to that muscle. So, to slim down your thighs you cycle, or to flatten your stomach you do sit-ups. Unfortunately, the body does not work like this. You cannot choose where you would like the fat to come from when you work out. Exercise stimulates a general rather than a specific use of fat through hormones delivered in the bloodstream to the whole body. Exercise will, however, build lean tissue, which influences the metabolic rate (see Myth 8, opposite). Strengthening certain areas, such as the abdominals and the hamstrings, also improves posture, and this in itself has a positive effect on your appearance.

5 Some diets target weight from one body area, such as the hips

This idea could be part of Myth 4. Unfortunately the theory doesn't add up and it is about as possible as emptying one side of a bottle.

6 Grapefruit and egg (substitute any food) is a magic combination for weight loss

"One-food-centered" diets are based on the idea that particular foods, or combinations of food, magically burn off fat. The theory is that the process of digesting certain foods requires more calories than they contain. You can undoubtedly lose weight fast on diets like this; they are simply very-low-calorie diets that border dangerously on starvation. You just won't lose the weight permanently. Apart from being repetitious and boring, these diets seriously lack nutrients, they slow down the metabolism, and provide very little energy.

7 The body cannot digest certain foods at the same time

This food "combining" theory is based on the idea that the digestive enzymes that break down protein and carbohydrates neutralize each other, leaving undigested foods to ferment in the gut, become toxic, and lead to obesity and constipation. If this were true, malnutrition rather than obesity would result. Medical opinion is that this type of diet only works by making the dieter monitor the quality and quantity of food they eat.

8 My metabolism is so slow, I can't lose weight

Everyone claims a friend who "eats like a horse and never gains weight," but scientists are still looking for this person. Depending on age and gender, we all burn food at about the same rate. This is because metabolic rate is linked to lean tissue; women naturally have less muscle and more fat than men, and muscle tends to decrease with age. Muscle burns fuel faster than fat, because it is a working part of the body – fat is just something we carry around. Dramatic weight loss through dieting depletes muscle mass, lowering your metabolic rate. The body learns to survive on fewer calories and, after the diet, healthy amounts of food become surplus to requirements and are stored as fat, so weight is quickly regained.

9 Wearing plastic or sweat gear helps weight loss

Forcing yourself to sweat makes you lose water, not fat. Water is essential to life, and you can drink as much as you like – it contains no calories and no fat.

10 Exercise is a useless way to lose weight: you have to burn 3,500 calories to lose just 1lb/0.45kg of fat

It is true that 1lb (0.45kg) of fat is worth about 3,500 calories. If you are used to starvation diets where the scales show a loss of five times this amount in a week, you might be disheartened. But the only way you can lose that much "weight" in a week is by losing muscle and water, and all the evidence shows it will return very quickly. Combining exercising with dieting means that more of the weight you lose will be from fat. Remember, the scales don't tell the whole truth: muscle is heavier than fat. 1lb (0.45kg) of fat takes up 31 cubic inches (508 cubic cm) of space – the size of a cabbage. 1lb (0.45kg) of muscle takes up only 25 cubic inches (410 cubic cm). If you replaced 5lb (2.25kg) of fat with 5lb (2.25kg) of muscle, you would weigh the same but would be around 30 cubic inches (492 cubic cm) smaller. Think about it.

The Facts

There is no magic formula for weight loss. You cannot lose weight without creating a "calorie deficit" – burning more calories as energy than you take in as food. In theory, you can choose one of three ways to do this: eat less, exercise more, or combine the two by eating a little less while exercising a little more. When the facts are laid out, the choice is obvious.

In contrast to all the myths about weight loss, there is one central fact:

Combining a reduced intake of food that is high in carbohydrates and low in fat with an appropriate exercise program is the only way to lose body fat and lose it permanently.

A diet high in carbohydrates will give you plenty of energy to exercise. The benefits of exercise are two-fold: it burns fat as a fuel and at the same time maintains muscle mass, so that your metabolic rate remains high despite the fact that you are losing weight. This method of losing weight may not be as seductive as the "lose weight fast" diets, but it really is the closest you will ever get to a magic formula for permanent weight loss.

The practical method

No doctor would recommend weight loss of more than 1–2lbs (0.45–1kg) per week. 1lb (0.45kg) of fat represents about 3,500 calories. This may seem a vast amount, but if the calorie deficit needed to lose it is spread over seven days, your daily deficit will be no more than 500 calories. By combining the right type of exercise with the right type of diet, you can achieve this quite easily without either starving yourself or killing yourself in the gym.

It may seem a slow process, but with this method you can be sure that you will be losing fat rather than muscle and water, and you can be sure that the weight will stay off. And bear in mind that 1lb (0.45kg) of fat is equal to 31 cubic inches (508 cubic cm) of body mass. Over 10 weeks, you could lose a massive 310 cubic inches (5,080 cubic cm) of fat. That is a lot of fat. Losing 1lb (0.45kg) of fat

weekly requires a calorie deficit of 500 calories a day. You can achieve this in the following way:

■ Decrease the energy you take in by 250 calories a day. The easiest way to do this is to stick to foods that are high in carbohydrates and low in fat (see pages 38 – 39). Fat has over twice the calories of carbohydrates, so cutting down on fat is the simplest and healthiest way to reduce calories. Carbohydrates are the body's essential fuel and, since you will be eating more of them, you won't feel weak and hungry. Complex carbohydrates release energy gradually, keeping the blood-sugar level constant, so you also will not suffer from sugar cravings.

■ At the same time, increase the energy you use every day by 250 calories. This can be achieved with 30 minutes of moderate aerobic exercise, such as cycling or jogging, or an hour's brisk walk. However unfit you feel, you can embark on an exercise program that will build up safely to achieve this (see page 55).

The benefits of losing weight in this way are numerous:

High energy A high-carbohydrate diet is high in energy, while low-calorie diets deliver exactly what they promise: low energy. A diet that leaves you weak and hungry leaves you open to temptation and usually results in the body's self-defense mechanism – binging.

Weight loss is permanent A diet high in carbohydrates won't leave you feeling lethargic and will give you enough energy to exercise. This will ensure that weight stays off, as opposed to the result of quick-fix diets, which guarantees that you'll regain weight just as quickly as you lost it.

Body fat is substantially decreased This method compares well with shorter diets of calorie restriction alone which have been shown to result in temporary weight loss, mainly from muscle and water, with only a slight decrease in fat.

Exercise re-educates the body Natural appetite cues are reprogrammed in those who exercise; in contrast, the appetite of an inactive person tends to "freewheel." If a program of weight loss includes exercise, there is less reliance on reducing calories, so there is less hunger and less temptation.

Muscle mass is maintained Aerobic exercise retains muscle mass, while fat is burned as a fuel, so your metabolic rate remains high.

Significant health benefits Unique benefits are achieved by increasing exercise and reducing fat. These include a reduced risk of several obesity-linked diseases that can endanger the heart. Weight-bearing exercise also maintains bone mass and helps guard against osteoporosis in old age.

Exercise releases endorphins These hormones with a "feel-good factor" give a sense of increased well-being. Exercise also provides an outlet from the stresses of everyday life and leaves you feeling physically and mentally refreshed. You will also benefit from the sense of actively contributing to your weight loss.

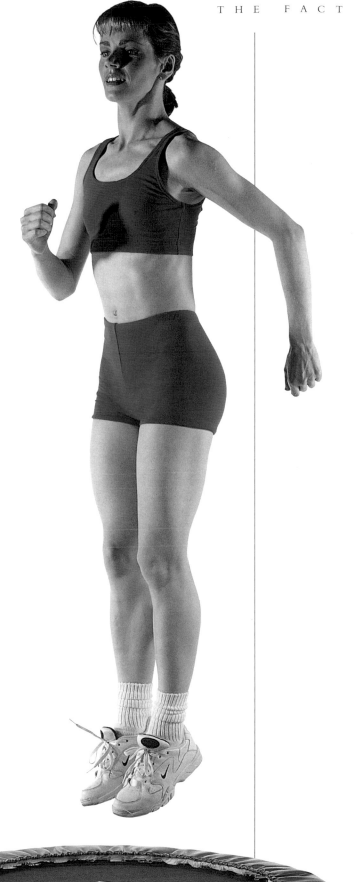

Using Energy

The muscles make up almost half of the body mass. There are over 660 different muscles in the human body, and even at rest they account for about 20% of the average daily energy you use. During all-out exercise this can increase by a hundredfold. The more exercise you do, the more energy the muscles burn.

Fuel for life

Although energy is usually associated with exercise, you don't use it only when you are on the go. Just as a car burns fuel even when the engine is idling, your body uses energy even when you are asleep simply in order to stay alive. Energy is not conjured up from thin air: it comes from your daily diet. The food you eat goes through a digestive process in which the useful parts are extracted and the waste expelled. Anything beyond what you need gets stored for future use.

Storing energy

Muscles are made up of 75% protein and 20% water. They are dense and compact: 1lb (0.45kg) of muscle takes up over 6 cubic inches (98 cubic cm) less room than 1lb (0.45kg) of fat. In the short term, a limited amount of carbohydrates can be stored in the muscles. Unfortunately, the only long-term storage system the body has is fat. Its capacity to store fat is practically unlimited, and fat is the ultimate destination of any food that is surplus to requirements. The average person has 2,000 calories' worth of carbohydrates stored, compared to about 80,000 calories' worth of fat. That's enough carbohydrates to run 20 miles, and more than enough fat to run from New York to Chicago.

Burning fat: the problem

It may seem hard to believe, but the body *prefers* to use fat for energy. It likes to save the carbohydrates to feed the brain, which needs around 4oz (120g) daily – the sugar in ten apples. We worry, quite rightly, when the brain is starved of oxygen, yet people often go on diets that starve the brain of sugar.

The body would like to use fat, and it has vast stores available. So why is obesity such a problem? First, because technology has eliminated most of the fat-burning activities from modern life: we can have clean clothes at the touch of a button and rarely walk anywhere. We're left with time on our hands and, as a direct consequence, flab on our hips. At the same time, food is cheaper and more plentiful than ever, and we eat rich and fatty foods every day: we are simply eating more fat than we burn. The result is an alarming increase in obesity that is beginning to rival even smoking-related diseases as a cause of death.

The solution

The one method of weight control proven to be successful in the long term works because it doesn't try to ignore the laws of nature. By combining a high-carbohydrate, low-fat diet with the right type of exercise, you tackle both the major causes of obesity, and weight loss is permanent. Forget all of those miracle cures: when you see the facts laid out in front of you, you will find that they are too persuasive to ignore.

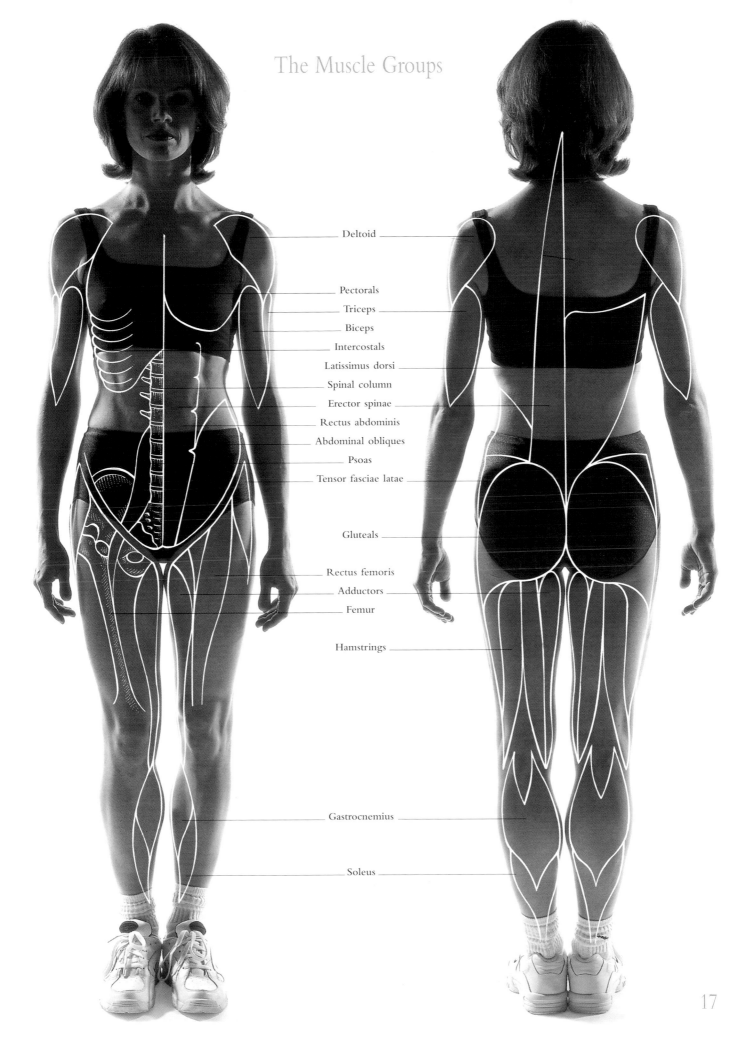

The Muscle Groups

Deltoid

Pectorals

Triceps

Biceps

Intercostals

Latissimus dorsi

Spinal column

Erector spinae

Rectus abdominis

Abdominal obliques

Psoas

Tensor fasciae latae

Gluteals

Rectus femoris

Adductors

Femur

Hamstrings

Gastrocnemius

Soleus

17

Diet or Exercise?

Most people who want to lose weight are more than willing to make whatever changes are necessary, but they aren't very clear on just what those changes should be. To lose weight in the long term, you need to consider diet, exercise, and weight control as three connected points of the same triangle.

Understanding the connection

Almost everyone has an opinion about losing weight. Some say it doesn't matter how much exercise you do: it's cutting down what you eat that counts. Others swear that increasing your activity is the only way to make a difference; the harder you work, the more weight you lose. As you can see below, neither argument in itself gives you the whole picture.

Diet

You will lose weight if you consistently eat less food than your body needs, and it might look quite impressive on the scales.

But diet without exercise makes you lose muscle and water, not fat, and within weeks the weight is bound to be back.

Exercise

Exercise is very effective at burning calories, and fat is a vast source of stored energy that can potentially be used as fuel.

However, if you continue to eat more fat than you need, the fat that you have lost will soon be back.

Weight control

It has been proven repeatedly that, although you can lose weight through diet or exercise, the best way to reduce body fat permanently is to combine the right exercise (see opposite) with a low-fat, high-carbohydrate diet.

The relationship between diet, exercise, and weight control

What is Exercise?

Every weekend, the parks are full of Sunday joggers attempting to run their way to a better figure. They go all out for as long as they can – a few minutes at the most – and are then forced to stop until they get their breath back again. They understand the need to exercise but are going about it the wrong way.

The two types of exercise

"Exercise" can describe absolutely any physical activity, from walking the dog to running a marathon. Yet, however sedate or strenuous the exercise might be, the body truly recognizes only two types: "aerobic" and "anaerobic." Which type it is depends on two factors: intensity (how hard you work) and duration (how long the work lasts).

Intensity and duration

In short bursts, we can produce a considerable amount of power. Most of us could manage a fair pace if it meant the difference between catching the bus or being forced to wait for the next one. World-class sprinters run the 400 meters in well under a minute. Yet even with years of training, they can't continue at full speed for much longer than this. It is simply the way the human body works. We are not designed to keep up intense effort over a long period of time, and pushing the body to the limit means that we very soon run out of steam.

While a high degree of effort can be sustained only in activity that lasts up to a minute or two, if the effort is reduced we can keep exercising for hours. We all know from experience that, whatever the activity, be it digging the garden or dancing the night away, the less effort we put in, the longer we can continue.

The length of time we can keep going during exercise is directly related to how hard we work. If exercise is so high in intensity that it limits duration, it is called "anaerobic" exercise, whereas if it is lower in intensity and sustainable, it is called "aerobic" exercise (see pages 20 – 21).

The effects of intensity versus duration

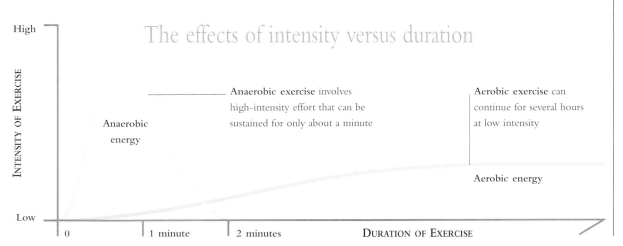

Anaerobic energy

Anaerobic exercise involves high-intensity effort that can be sustained for only about a minute

Aerobic exercise can continue for several hours at low intensity

Aerobic energy

High

INTENSITY OF EXERCISE

Low

0   1 minute   2 minutes   DURATION OF EXERCISE

Which Type of Exercise?

Once you have accepted that exercise plays an important part in weight loss, you need to know which type of exercise you should do to derive the maximum benefit. To burn body fat, you must exercise at low to moderate intensity for at least 20 minutes.

LACTIC ACID

The anaerobic system is sometimes known as the "lactic acid system." Lactic acid is blamed for sore muscles and cramps, and is seen as a waste product. In fact, it is vital to both energy systems and is formed even when we rest. It is a problem only during anaerobic exercise, when it builds up in muscle until we are forced to ease off or stop.

The two energy systems

Just as there are two types of exercise, the body has two systems for producing the energy that exercise requires. These are called the anaerobic and aerobic systems. Both systems burn carbohydrates, but only one of them eventually burns fat. Unless your exercise is fueled by the aerobic system, all the sweating in the world won't help. Very demanding exercise might keep you fit, but it doesn't necessarily keep you thin.

The short-term (anaerobic) system

Anaerobic literally means "without air." During anaerobic exercise – intense exercise lasting about a minute – the demand for energy is either so sudden or so great that the heart is unable to pump enough oxygen to the working muscles.

Because there is insufficient oxygen in the muscles, the body must find another way of producing energy – one that doesn't involve oxygen. It does this through a series of steps that break down the energy from carbohydrates. All anaerobic exercise is fueled by the anaerobic system, and it burns carbohydrates, not fat. When you start to exercise, your heart begins to beat faster in response to the increased need for oxygen. Until enough oxygen is available to the muscles, all energy needs to be supplied anaerobically.

The anaerobic system therefore acts as the gateway to all activity, and the consequent buildup of lactic acid (see side panel, left) explains the "heavy legs" that make exercise seem so tiring in the beginning. When oxygen reaches the muscles, the lactic acid is recycled.

ANAEROBIC EXERCISE

High intensity, short duration

- *Running up the stairs*
- *Sprinting*
- *Push-starting the car*

The long-term (aerobic) system

Aerobic means "with air." All oxygen is delivered around the body in blood pumped by the heart. The aerobic system can function only when the energy demand is low enough for the heart to supply the muscles with sufficient oxygen – the sort of exercise you do when you are breathing hard but not gasping for breath.

Aerobic exercise is fueled predominantly by the aerobic system. Both carbohydrates and fat can supply fuel for this system, but when exercise lasts for less than 20 minutes, carbohydrates will always provide the fuel. Only when the exercise goes beyond this can fat contribute to the supply.

AEROBIC EXERCISE:

Low to moderate intensity, long duration

- *Walking the dog*
- *Jogging*
- *Cycling to stores*

□ Anaerobic exercise

□ Aerobic exercise

□ Aerobic endurance exercise

Aerobic endurance

There is a variation of aerobic exercise called "aerobic endurance exercise." This is when exercise continues at a low level over a long period of time. It is only during this type of activity that fat is broken down and used as the main source of energy.

Fat molecules are difficult to break down, and it takes the body a while to "gear up" its fat-burning cycle. This is why exercise designed specifically to burn fat is sometimes called "endurance" exercise. Unless your workout is relatively low in intensity and lasts over 20 minutes, the body has no choice but to burn stored carbohydrates instead. Carbohydrates can fuel both energy systems, but fat can be burned only in aerobic endurance exercise. If you want to get rid of excess body fat once and for all, this type of exercise is, without a doubt, the best way to do it. Although 20 minutes' or more exercise may sound like a lot, don't be put off. The whole point of aerobic endurance exercise is that the intensity is low enough to be easily sustained over a long period of time.

Fat doesn't fuel all long-term exercise. When high-intensity exercise continues over a long time, carbohydrates provide the energy – marathon runners are fueled primarily by the pasta they eat in the days before the race. You can store enough carbohydrates to provide the energy for about one and a half hours' of high-intensity exercise. Because there are several endurance events that last longer than this, there is a time when carbohydrate storage will run out: this is commonly called "hitting the wall." Neither energy process happens independently of the other, and they can and do overlap. The body switches between the systems according to the demands you make of it.

LIMITED LUNG CAPACITY

Every healthy person can do aerobic endurance exercise. Some use "limited lung capacity" as an excuse if they get seriously out of breath, but the limiting factor is usually the heart's inefficiency through lack of training. The heart is a muscle that, like any other, can be improved with training. An individual's lung capacity is more or less fixed.

AEROBIC ENDURANCE EXERCISE:

Low intensity, over 20 minutes

- *An hour's walk*
- *A 30-minute swim*
- *A country hike*

Reading Your Heart Rate

If you want to lose body fat permanently, you need to use it as a fuel in aerobic endurance exercise (see page 21). Your watch tells you how long you are working – the endurance element – and it can also help you check that you aren't working too hard.

Hitting the right intensity

You find out how hard you are working by measuring your heart rate. During exercise your heart rate goes up; the harder you work, the faster the heart beats. Everyone has a maximum heart rate – the fastest it can possibly beat. Calculating how close your heart rate is to its maximum during exercise enables you to check the intensity of your workout.

Reading your heart rate

Your training heart rate must be measured during exercise, but you may find it useful to take a few practice readings while resting. It takes time to become proficient, and initial attempts may be a little far-fetched.

1 *Find your pulse either on the underside of your wrist, or on the side of your neck. Use your first two fingers, not the thumb – it has its own pulse, which can distort the accuracy of a reading. You may need to make a brief stop, but take your pulse immediately.*

2 *Start counting your pulse when the second hand of your watch reaches a given point, and count the beats over the next six seconds.*

3 *Multiply this number by 10 to work out the number of beats in 60 seconds and you have the beats per minute (BPM). This is your heart rate. You can test the accuracy by counting the beats over 30 seconds and multiplying them by 2 to see if you get the same result.*

EXAMPLE:

- *The second hand of your watch is at 35 seconds.*
- *You count 12 heartbeats by the time it reaches the 41 seconds mark.*
- *Multiply 12 by 10 and you find your heart rate is 120 beats per minute.*

Using a heart-rate monitor

You can also check your heart rate using an electronic heart-rate monitor. This will give an accurate readout of your heart rate throughout exercise. Different models are available, but you need only the most basic (and the cheapest).

1 Strap the transmitter band of the monitor around your chest, directly next to your skin. This will relay information to the monitor.

2 Strap the monitor, which resembles a digital watch, to your wrist. The display will show you a constant reading of your heart rate.

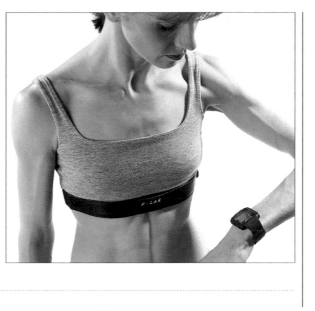

Your maximum heart rate

To calculate if you are working at the right intensity, you also need to know your maximum heart rate. Although there are tests to measure this, they aren't necessary unless you have a heart problem; instead, it can be estimated. As you get older, the maximum rate at which your heart can beat decreases, so the age-based formula on the right works as a guideline.

Your age-predicted maximum heart rate = (220 minus your age)

- *If you are 18 years old, your age-predicted maximum will be:*   *220 - 18 = 202 BPM*
- *If you are 25 years old:*   *220 - 25 = 195 BPM*
- *If you are 35 years old:*   *220 - 35 = 185 BPM*
- *If you are 50 years old:*   *220 - 50 = 170 BPM*
- *If you are 65 years old:*   *220 - 65 = 155 BPM*

Target zones for different types of exercise

In anaerobic exercise

Your heart is working faster than 85% of its maximum heart rate (see above):

Running up the stairs

Sprinting

Push-starting the car

- *If you are 18 years old: at least 171 BPM*
- *If you are 25 years old: at least 165 BPM*
- *If you are 35 years old: at least 157 BPM*
- *If you are 50 years old: at least 144 BPM*
- *If you are 65 years old: at least 131 BPM*

In aerobic exercise

Your heart is working between 60% and 85% of its maximum heart rate (see above):

Walking the dog

Jogging

Cycling to stores

- *If you are 18 years old: between 121 and 171 BPM*
- *If you are 25 years old: between 117 and 165 BPM*
- *If you are 35 years old: between 111 and 157 BPM*
- *If you are 50 years old: between 102 and 144 BPM*
- *If you are 65 years old: between 93 and 131 BPM*

In aerobic endurance exercise

Your heart is working between 60% and 70% of its maximum heart rate for at least 20 minutes (see above):

An hour's walk

30 minutes of cycling

A country hike

- *If you are 18 years old: between 121 and 141 BPM*
- *If you are 25 years old: between 117 and 136 BPM*
- *If you are 35 years old: between 111 and 129 BPM*
- *If you are 50 years old: between 102 and 119 BPM*
- *If you are 65 years old: between 93 and 108 BPM*

CAUTION

If you have a family history of heart problems, check with your doctor before starting any exercise program.

Energy
for Life
Total Nutrition Guide

Many of us have, at some time in our lives, attempted the regime of semi-starvation called the "low-calorie diet." You eat less than you need, hoping to burn excess fat. This is a short-term solution to a long-term problem: sustained, healthy weight control lies in balancing the carbohydrates, protein, and fat you eat.

But how can you translate this theory to the food on your plate? While traditional diets tell you to obsessively count the calories in each meal, my method is much simpler. By understanding the essential food groups, you can learn to balance every meal. Since doing this, I have been neither hungry nor lacking in energy, and my struggle to control my weight has become a thing of the past.

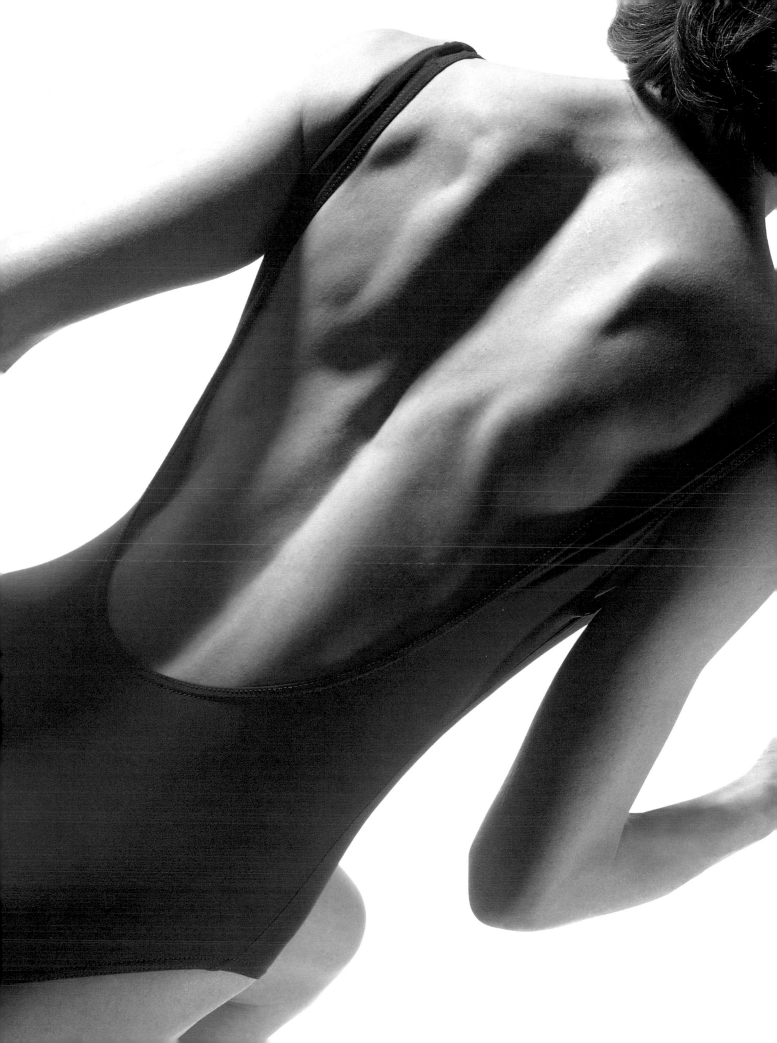

The Lowdown on Calories

For most people, "going on a diet" means counting and cutting calories. Filled with optimism and determination, they clear the refrigerator of anything vaguely appetizing and load it up with foods that boast they promote weight loss as part of a calorie-controlled diet.

What is a calorie?

You can certainly lose weight on a calorie-controlled diet, although for how long is open to question. Unfortunately, you'll also lose the most important thing that calories supply: energy. Despite years of obsessively counting them, most dieters are still not very clear on exactly what a calorie is. Before you decide to cut them, it might be a good idea to find out.

Cutting energy

Most of the food you buy, (and certainly all the packaged food) tells you how many calories it contains. Imported foods will use one or more of three words: "kcals," "kjoules," or "energy." The last of these provides the clue: the calorie content of food doesn't indicate how fat you'll get if you eat that food. It tells you how much energy it will provide. This is why cutting calories inevitably means cutting energy; the two terms are interchangeable. In nutritional terms, calories measure the energy provided by the food you eat to "heat" or fuel your body. "Calorie expenditure" is the amount of energy you use.

If that were the end of the story, you could argue that the more calories you ate, the more energy you would have and, in a way, you would be right. You would certainly have a lot of potential energy, but recent research shows that you are unlikely to use it. We burn far fewer calories every week than our grandparents did, and our lifestyles rarely include the sort of long-term activity that burns fat. Most of the energy we use comes from carbohydrates. Unfortunately, less useful calories don't just disappear. You either use them or you store them, and the only long-term storage system we have is body fat.

Where do calories come from?

Carbohydrates, protein, and fat provide all the energy your body uses, but the recipe for good health has three other essential ingredients; vitamins, minerals, and water. The absence of any one of these six elements would eventually lead to illness and, in the long term, would prove fatal. Vitamins, minerals, and water play an important part in just about everything that goes on in your body, but, contrary to popular belief, they do not supply energy; they are calorie-free, and energy comes only with calories.

All calories come from four sources: carbohydrates, protein, fat, and alcohol. Alcohol contributes very little to sound nutrition yet at the same time manages to supply a considerable number of fairly useless calories. If you're trying to lose weight, you should try to drink as little alcohol as possible.

Although most foods can be categorized as mainly one type or another, there are very few which are uniquely carbohydrate, protein, or fat. In most cases, the calories come from two or three sources. To control your weight, it's not the number of calories you should be watching, but where they come from. Some calories are just more useful than others.

How many calories do you need?

Your body uses energy simply to stay alive. The resting metabolic rate tells you how many calories your body would use if you spent the entire day lying down. To get an idea of how much energy you really use, you need to add on the energy required in day-to-day living – getting up and going to work, for instance – and the energy you use in eating and digesting food. These three elements make up your total daily energy expenditure.

Survival tactics

It is highly unlikely that, as an adult, your body could maintain itself, even at rest, on fewer than 1,200 calories. If you try to survive on less than this, you will be hard pushed to get all the nutrients you require for long-term health. In addition to this, taking in fewer calories than your body needs encourages it to break down protein (your muscles) to supply energy. Because it influences your metabolism, depleting muscle mass leads to a lowering of the metabolic rate.

Dramatic weight loss through diet alone has been proven to have a serious (and sustained) effect on metabolism, above and beyond the effect of losing lean tissue. The body is designed to survive famine, even when it is self-inflicted. In severe diets, the metabolic rate can be depressed by as much as 45% as the body becomes more energy efficient, slowing down its systems to enable it to survive on fewer calories. It's a bit like driving a car that is low on gas. If you want to make it last until the nearest gas station, you have no option but to drive very slowly. The lower the speed, the less fuel you burn. As your metabolic rate goes down, the body uses less energy, and you will find it harder to lose weight, however little you eat. Regular exercise, on the other hand, can raise your metabolic rate by maintaining, and even increasing, muscle mass.

ESTIMATING YOUR RESTING METABOLIC RATE (RMR)

You can estimate your RMR by multiplying your weight in pounds by 10 (1lb = 0.45kg)

- *If you weigh 130lb, your RMR will be approximately 1,300 calories: 130 X 10 = 1,300*

Remember, the resting metabolic rate is not your ideal calorie intake; it only tells you how many calories you would need to lie in bed all day.

How the body uses energy

Between 60 and 75% of the energy you use in a day is taken up in staying alive. Physical activity – working, shopping, or exercising – accounts for a further 15 – 30%, depending on how active you are. A small amount of energy is used in digesting food. By far the easiest way to increase your energy expenditure is to add on exercise – lumberjacks and endurance athletes use twice as much energy every day as the average adult.

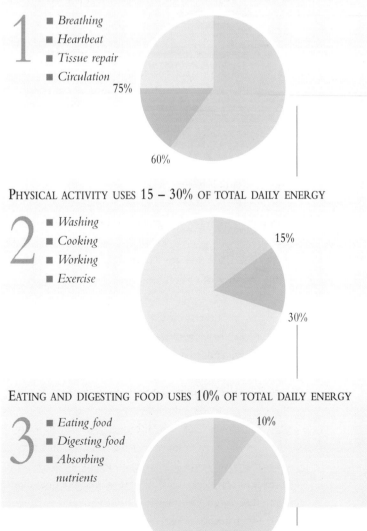

RESTING METABOLIC RATE USES 60 – 75% OF TOTAL DAILY ENERGY

1
- *Breathing*
- *Heartbeat*
- *Tissue repair*
- *Circulation*

75%

60%

PHYSICAL ACTIVITY USES 15 – 30% OF TOTAL DAILY ENERGY

2
- *Washing*
- *Cooking*
- *Working*
- *Exercise*

15%

30%

EATING AND DIGESTING FOOD USES 10% OF TOTAL DAILY ENERGY

3
- *Eating food*
- *Digesting food*
- *Absorbing nutrients*

10%

Carbohydrates

This is a catchall term for starchy and sweet foods, from pasta to sugar cubes. Carbohydrates are the major fuel for all physical activity, and that doesn't just mean the kind of exercise that athletes do – it includes running for the bus as well. A low-carbohydrate diet leads to low energy, which leads to low activity – this is how weight begins to creep up.

What do they do?

■ Stored in the liver and muscles as glycogen, carbohydrates serve as a major energy source for all activity.
■ Carbohydrates are the main fuel of the central nervous system (which includes the brain).
■ They are an essential part of the fat-burning process, serving as a primer: if carbohydrates are not present, fat cannot be broken down completely.
■ They provide 4 calories of energy per gram.

Where are they found?

Nature has given us three types of carbohydrates, all of which can be called "unrefined."

Simple carbohydrates

Often referred to collectively as "simple sugars," these include glucose (a sugar that occurs naturally in foods such as fruit), fructose (another natural sugar in fruit), lactose (present in milk, including breast milk), and sucrose (found in sugarcane).

Complex carbohydrates

These are also known as starches. Plants store carbohydrates as starch, which is found in rice, flour, and potatoes. Starch is made up of a chain of simple sugars linked together, which means it is slower to break down, and releases its energy over a longer period.

GOOD SOURCES OF UNREFINED CARBOHYDRATES

CHOOSE WHOLE-GRAIN VARIETIES WHENEVER POSSIBLE.

PASTA

BREAD

BREAKFAST CEREALS

GRAINS, SUCH AS RICE, COUSCOUS, WHEAT, AND CORN

BEANS

FRUIT

DRIED FRUIT

POTATOES AND OTHER ROOT VEGETABLES

DAILY REQUIREMENT
Unrefined carbohydrate foods should make up more than half of the food on your plate.

Dietary fiber

An integral part of most unrefined carbohydrates, fiber is found in the cell walls of vegetables, fruit, beans, and whole-grain cereals. Most fiber cannot be digested by humans, but it is still extremely beneficial. It provides bulk, which makes you feel full, naturally limiting the amount you eat at any one time. Fiber also acts as a binding agent and speeds up the passage of food through the intestines. In this way, fiber helps to guard against gastrointestinal disease and colon cancer.

Refined sugar

Man has managed to introduce a fourth carbohydrate into the diet. Refined sugar, such as table sugar, is not found in nature, which is a good indication of just how much the body needs it. It is used to add sweetness to confectionery, cakes, cookies, and a good deal of supposedly "savory" food. It provides plenty of calories, and therefore plenty of energy, but contributes no nutritional value to your diet, because refined carbohydrates are stripped of all their vitamins, minerals, and fiber. Refined sugar releases its energy very quickly, triggering an abrupt insulin response that can lead to light-headedness and "blood sugar jitters" (see page 54). After an initial high, your energy levels feel lower than they did *before* you ate, until they eventually stabilize.

Unrefined vs. refined carbohydrates

Unrefined carbohydrates, such as whole-wheat bread, whole-wheat pasta, whole-grain cereals, brown rice, and fruit, provide valuable vitamins and minerals along with energy. The process of refining whole-wheat flour into white, for example, strips it of nutrients, leaving little else apart from calories. This is one of the reasons why unrefined carbohydrates are a much healthier choice.

Weight control

As well as providing vitamins and minerals, unrefined carbohydrates contribute fiber to the diet, which is an important factor in appetite control (and in curbing weight gain). I find it impossible to overeat on unrefined carbohydrates – they are almost self-limiting. You feel full much sooner from a meal of unrefined carbohydrates than from one based on protein, fat, or refined sugar, so you can satisfy your appetite without overloading on calories. Baked potatoes, for example, have the same amount of energy/calories as an iced doughnut, but while doughnuts are mainly sugar and fat, potatoes are high in fiber and complex carbohydrates. You might be able to eat two or three doughnuts, but you would be hard-pushed to manage more than one large baked potato. Foods high in unrefined carbohydrates are not only more filling, they are also usually lower in fat.

CARBOHYDRATE FOODS TO LIMIT IN YOUR DIET

SUGAR
(WHITE & BROWN)

CANDY

CHOCOLATE

CAKES

COOKIES

SUGARY DRINKS

JAM

HONEY

SYRUPS

Protein

The role of protein – maintaining and repairing tissue – cannot be fulfilled by any other nutrient, but there is no benefit at all from eating excessive amounts. Protein won't give you more energy or stronger muscles, and it can be detrimental rather than beneficial to health.

In fact, you need much less protein than often imagined.

LOW-FAT SOURCES OF PROTEIN

Remove the fat or skin from meat and poultry, and use a low-fat method of cooking, such as steaming or broiling, to prepare food.

■

VERY LEAN MEAT

■

FISH

■

SKINLESS POULTRY

■

TOFU

■

PEAS & BEANS

■

LOW-FAT DAIRY PRODUCTS

■

SMALL AMOUNTS OF PROTEIN ARE ALSO FOUND IN BREAD, PASTA, & BREAKFAST CEREALS

DAILY REQUIREMENT

Protein should make up 10 – 20% of the daily diet.

What does it do?

■ Protein maintains, repairs, and builds the living tissue in the body, but, despite popular opinion, you don't increase muscle bulk by eating extra protein.
■ It is the main component of muscles, tendons, and ligaments.
■ When you don't eat sufficient amounts of carbohydrates, protein can be converted to glucose to provide energy for both the muscles and the brain. The use of protein for energy takes precedence over its foremost task, maintaining tissues, which means injuries and wounds are slower to heal.
■ Protein provides 4 calories of energy per gram.

Where is it found?

Protein is present in most foods. It is made up of several amino acids, the building blocks of living tissue. You need around 20 different amino acids, and they can be split into two categories. Eight of them (nine for children) cannot be made within the body, so you need to get them from what you eat. These eight are known as "essential" amino acids. This does not mean that the remaining twelve are not necessary – they are all essential for health – but they can be manufactured in the body from the essential amino acids in your diet.

Protein quality

Foods contain amino acids in varying proportions, and the quality of a protein is measured by how closely the amino acids match the human body's requirements. The closer the match, the more efficiently it can be used. The amino acids in animal proteins, such as eggs, milk, cheese, meat, poultry, and fish, are very close to human requirements. They are said to have a high biological value and are described as "complete" proteins. Protein from plant sources is not generally as well-matched, but since meals are usually based around a variety of foods, such as bread with cheese, rice with lentils, or vegetables with pasta, it is not difficult to get a well-balanced mix of amino acids, even if you don't eat meat. You don't need to balance the amino acids in every meal, but the greater the variety of protein sources in your diet, the better.

The best sources of protein

Protein is present, to some degree, in almost everything you eat; the only foods that contain absolutely no protein are vegetable and nut oils and refined table sugar. It is not particularly high in most fruit and vegetables, although foods from other plant sources, such as beans, whole-grain cereals, rice, and pasta, contain a significant amount of protein. Vegetarians and vegans who eat a wide variety of these foods should not be protein deficient – especially if they eat soybeans, which are as high in protein as eggs and cheese.

The great protein myth

Despite the wealth of sensible information available, there is a persistent misunderstanding about protein and how much is really needed. It should make up only between 10–20% of what you eat, but, since the heyday of the high-protein/low-carbohydrate diet in the Seventies, broiled steak and lean chicken have been the cornerstone of the dieter's plate. Potatoes and pasta continue to be seen as no-go areas for anyone watching their weight. Yet, while many high-carbohydrate foods contain only a trace of fat, high-protein foods are often a source of hidden fat. Even lean beef derives about 50% of its calories from fat and the other half from protein. Although protein is certainly an important part of the diet – we couldn't do without it – according to recent research, when the most popular types of diet were compared, the high-protein/low-carbohydrate diet was the only one for which no advantages could be found.

In a high-protein regime, where you restrict the amount of carbohydrates you eat, the body is forced to use protein as an energy source. The stores of carbohydrates (about 2,000 calories' worth) are used up in about 24 hours. The brain needs a constant level of sugar in the blood, and when it isn't provided in the diet, the body supplies it by converting protein to glucose. This diverts protein from its main task of repairing and maintaining tissue. In extreme cases of starvation, the body turns to its protein stores – the muscles – to provide energy. Loss of muscle mass through dieting can lead to a lowering of the metabolic rate and can be dangerous.

Weight control

Today, two-thirds of the protein we eat is derived from animal produce; 70 years ago, it came equally from plants and animals. Since meat products contain not only protein but also fat, many of us are taking in much higher levels of saturated fat than we need. It is hardly surprising that up to a quarter of adults in the Western world are considered to be overweight, and that heart disease is now a major cause of death in most industrialized nations.

HIGH-FAT SOURCES OF PROTEIN

■

FATTY MEAT

■

EGGS

■

WHOLE-MILK DAIRY PRODUCTS

■

NUTS

31

Fat

As much as we love to hate it, fat is suprisingly palatable; it adds flavor and texture to the food we eat. A little fat is vital for good health, but since fat is present in most foods, especially those high in protein, it creeps into your diet more than you realize. Unless you eat a very limited diet, you should get enough fat without trying.

What does it do?

■ Certain fatty acids are essential: they cannot be made in the body, but they are needed to help form cell walls and for growth, sexual reproduction, and skin maintenance.
■ It carries the fat-soluble vitamins A, D, E, and K.
■ Fat is important as a fuel in light and moderate long-term activity.
■ At 9 calories per gram, fat provides over twice as much energy as carbohydrates.

Where is it found?

There are two types of fat: saturated and unsaturated. Unsaturated fat is no lower in calories than any other fat. But it's a better choice, because saturated fat can raise blood cholesterol levels, which can lead to heart disease. For good health, at least two-thirds of the fat you eat should be unsaturated.

Saturated fat

Found mainly in animal and dairy products like butter, lard, cheese, fatty meat, eggs, and whole milk, saturated fat tends to be solid at room temperature; the firmer the fat, the more saturated it is. There are some exceptions to this: palm and coconut oil are high in saturated fat despite being liquid.

Unsaturated fat

There are two types of unsaturated fat: polyunsaturated and monounsaturated, and they are usually liquid at room temperature. Olive oil is probably the best-known source of monounsaturated fat; other sources include canola oil and sesame oil. Polyunsaturated fat includes sunflower oil, soybean oil, safflower oil, corn oil, walnut oil, peanut oil, and fish oil. Replacing saturated with unsaturated fat can reduce the level of LDL, or "bad," cholesterol, the type that leads to narrowing of the arteries. The omega-3 fatty acids found in cold-water fish such as tuna, herring, mackerel, and sardines are thought to have a beneficial effect on health, lowering the risk of heart disease.

Hydrogenated fat

Most margarines and spreads contain a mixture of fats but advertise that they are "high in polyunsaturates." The process of hydrogenation, which makes liquid fats solid enough to be sold in a tub rather than a bottle, adds hydrogen, which converts unsaturated fat into saturated fat, making it less beneficial to health. Hydrogenated fat is also found in foods such as sausages, cookies, and cakes.

Cholesterol

A vital substance in the body, cholesterol is made by all animals, including humans. When your diet is high in saturated fat, the liver is stimulated to make more cholesterol than the body needs. The level of cholesterol in the blood goes up, and cholesterol-rich deposits are formed on the arteries that supply the heart with blood. This causes them to narrow and can eventually lead to a heart attack. Saturated fat has a more harmful effect than the cholesterol found in foods, but substituting unsaturated fats can help to lower blood cholesterol levels. Cholesterol is not found in vegetable foods.

Lowering your fat intake

There are two major reasons why the fat you eat should be kept to a minimum: it is bad for your health, and it leads to weight gain. Any excess food you eat will be stored as fat; however, fat is more easily converted to body fat than any other nutrient. The best way to lose weight is to replace fat with carbohydrate-rich foods. Many foods are now available in reduced or low-fat versions; some stores highlight items that are naturally low in fat. But beware: when fat is removed or reduced, it is often (not always) replaced with refined sugar. The list below gives alternatives that are no less filling but are much less fattening.

SOURCES OF SATURATED FAT

- FATTY CUTS OF MEAT
- MEAT PRODUCTS, SUCH AS SAUSAGES & PIES
- WHOLE-MILK DAIRY PRODUCTS
- BUTTER
- SOME MARGARINES
- PALM OIL
- COCONUT OIL
- COOKIES
- CAKES
- SAVORY SNACKS

CUT OUT:	REPLACE WITH:
Croissants	Bagels
Butter or margarine	Low-fat spread
Whole-milk dairy products	Low-fat dairy products
Cream or oil-based salad dressings	Yogurt-based or low-fat dressings
French fries	Potatoes, boiled or baked
Cheese or cream sauces	Vegetable-based sauces
Fried fish or meat	Broiled fish or meat
Fatty meat or sausages	Poultry without skin, lean cuts of meat
Candy, snacks, and chips	Fruit, rice cakes, vegetables

Vitamins & Minerals

An essential part of every process that happens in the body, these nutrients are vital for good health. Supplements are rarely necessary, because a varied diet normally provides all you need.

What do they do?

■ There are 13 known vitamins that play a vital role in most body processes. Whatever the ads say, vitamins and minerals do not supply energy: they mainly assist in the release of energy.

■ There are 22 known minerals that regulate body functions and provide structure in the formation of bones and teeth.

Where are they found?

Since the body cannot manufacture vitamins or minerals, these nutrients must be included in your diet. Vitamins are found in all fresh, raw food, but processing, overcooking, and storing food for long periods reduce the vitamin content. Lightly cooked food (steamed or broiled) is the best option. You need vitamins in very small amounts, and it is much better to get them as part of a healthy diet than through expensive supplements. Most minerals occur freely in nature: in water, topsoil, and below the Earth's surface. They are therefore found in the plants and animals we eat, and a varied, balanced diet should provide all the minerals you need.

Vitamins

There are two types of vitamins. Fat-soluble vitamins – A, D, E, and K – are stored in the body for long periods of time, so it takes months of deprivation before deficiency becomes a problem. Water-soluble vitamins – B complex and C – cannot be stored and must be included in your daily diet. Any excess is usually excreted in urine, although some can accumulate in the body. A balanced diet should provide all the

---

GOOD SOURCES OF VITAMINS & MINERALS

■

RAW FRUIT & VEGETABLES

■

LIGHTLY COOKED, FRESH OR FROZEN FRUIT & VEGETABLES

■

WHOLE-GRAIN CEREALS & GRAINS

■

LOW-FAT DAIRY PRODUCTS

■

BEANS & PEAS

■

LEAN MEAT

DAILY REQUIREMENT

Eat five or more different fruits and vegetables each day to ensure a good intake of vitamins and minerals. Choose fresh or frozen in preference to canned (see pages 38 – 39).

vitamins you need, but if you think you need a supplement, limit yourself to a multi-vitamin that provides the recommended daily amount. Diagnosing individual vitamin deficiencies is best left to your doctor, as overdoses can be toxic.

Minerals

A balanced diet should provide sufficient minerals, but particular attention should be paid to calcium and iron intake.

Calcium Vital for nerve transmission and blood clotting, calcium also gives bones their strength. If you eat insufficient calcium, the body steals calcium from the bones. This can lead to osteoporosis, a condition which makes the bones fragile and prone to fracture. Osteoporosis does affect men, but women are at greater risk, especially if they are very thin, eat insufficient calcium-rich foods, drink too much caffeine, or smoke. The female hormone estrogen, which has a protective effect on bone mass, is reduced after menopause. Women who do not menstruate regularly are also particularly vulnerable and should consult a doctor. The best defense against osteoporosis is to combine a good calcium intake with weight-bearing exercise, such as brisk walking, which stimulates bone formation. Women should try to maximize bone strength during their twenties.

Sources: Milk, dairy products (low-fat versions contain just as much), canned salmon and sardines (as long as you eat the bones), tofu, green leafy vegetables, and beans. You need about 800mg of calcium a day.

Iron Because this mineral is lost during menstruation, iron deficiency is fairly common in women. This is one of the instances where a doctor may prescribe a supplement.

Sources: Red meat, liver, egg yolk, green leafy vegetables, bread, beans, fortified breakfast cereals, and some dried fruit. The iron in non-meat produce is not easily absorbed by the body, but you can increase absorption by eating or drinking a source of vitamin C, such as a glass of orange juice, at the same time. A simple way to increase iron intake is to use unenameled, cast-iron skillets.

Salt Sweating causes the body to lose salt, but the need for added salt is probably more imagined than real. Most of us eat twice as much salt as we need. Excess sodium (a component of salt) can lead to high blood pressure, which in turn can increase the risk of strokes.

Sources: Watch out for added salt in smoked fish, savory snacks, and in many processed foods.

FOODS WITH A
REDUCED VITAMIN &
MINERAL CONTENT

■

FOOD STORED FOR
A LONG TIME

■

OVER-COOKED FOOD

■

FOOD KEPT WARM
FOR A LONG TIME

■

CANNED FOOD

■

PROCESSED FOOD

■

PEELED FRUIT &
VEGETABLES

■

REFINED FOOD

Water

Of the six components necessary for a healthy diet, water is probably the most overlooked. It contains no carbohydrates, protein, or fat – and therefore no calories – yet it is crucial for survival.

DRINKS THAT HYDRATE

▪

WATER

▪

FRUIT JUICE

▪

HERB TEAS

▪

FRUIT TEAS

▪

SKIM & LOW-FAT MILK

What does it do?

▪ It transports nutrients into and throughout the body, and it carries waste products out of the body.
▪ Water stabilizes body temperature.
▪ Essential for lubricating the joints, water also helps blood and other tissue fluids to flow freely.

Where is it found ?

Most of your daily intake of water comes from what you drink, but a significant amount is provided by food. Some foods, such as fruit and vegetables, contain a great deal of water; bananas, for example, are 75% water. Other foods, like butter, oil, cookies, and cakes, contain very little. A small amount of water is also produced by the body during the process of breaking down food for energy.

Tea, coffee, and many carbonated drinks contain caffeine, which is a diuretic and speeds up the loss of water, increasing dehydration. Drinks that are high in sugar aren't much help either, because they slow down the rate at which water can be absorbed from the stomach and put to use. Even fruit juices can be deceptively high in sugar. The most efficient drink for quenching thirst is also the most straightforward: cool, preferably not iced, water.

Fluid balance

You can last without food for several weeks, but you wouldn't survive for more than a few days without water. The amount of water you drink should balance the amount you use. An adult needs about 2 quarts (2.5 liters) – around eight glasses – of water a day; in hot weather, or during exercise, you obviously need more.

Despite its importance, very few people drink enough water. By the time you feel thirsty, the dehydration process is already well under way, and reaching for a drink that dehydrates makes the situation worse.

DAILY REQUIREMENT

An adult needs about 2 quarts (2.5 liters) of water a day. For every half hour of exercise, you should drink a glass of water.

Water loss

Water is lost from the body in several ways:

As urine When protein is broken down, it leaves a waste product called urea, which must be expelled from the body in urine. The more protein you eat, the more urea is produced. Since more water is then needed to flush away the urea, eating large quantities of protein can speed up dehydration.

As feces Made up of approximately 70% water, this accounts for a loss of about 4fl oz (100ml) of water a day. With diarrhea or vomiting, the fluid loss can increase to 4 quarts (5 liters), so fluid replacement is vital.

Through the skin To maintain body temperature, you continually lose a small amount of fluid, called insensible perspiration, through your skin without ever being aware of it. You also lose over 1 pint (600ml) of water every day in sweat – exercising in hot climates can produce up to 1 quart (1 liter) of sweat an hour.

From the lungs When you exhale, water is lost. You see it only in cold weather, when your breath forms a mist, but it is present whatever the temperature.

Losing water vs. losing weight

Water accounts for about two-thirds of your body weight. Getting rid of this water by sweating might seem like a good way to lose weight, but losing water is not the same as losing fat. If it were, the clothes you sweat in would feel greasy, not wet.

If you stand on the scales as soon as you finish exercising, a sweaty workout will look like a weight loss. But wait a few hours, drink a glass or two of water, and weigh yourself again: you will find that your weight is pretty much back to normal. It isn't a good idea to try to sweat yourself thin. First, it won't work – any weight loss will be only temporary; more importantly, losing even a small amount of water has serious health implications. It can affect blood pressure, temperature regulation, and coordination, and when coordination is impaired, you are at risk of injury.

It is not sweat itself, but the evaporation of sweat, that is the cooling mechanism of the body. In conditions of 100% humidity, the air is already saturated with as much water as it can hold, and sweat cannot evaporate. It simply rolls off the body, and the cooling effect is lost.

Wearing plastic (sweat or sauna) pants affects the efficiency of sweating. By preventing the evaporation of sweat, plastic pants simply inhibit your cooling system, and your body overheats. Body wraps in beauty salons work on the same principle; despite the miraculous claims for weight loss, the only thing you are losing is fluid. As soon as the body's water levels are replenished, you return to your original weight. Water loss doesn't affect body fat one little bit.

DRINKS THAT CONTAIN CAFFEINE

■

COFFEE

■

TEA

■

COLA

■

SOME ENERGY DRINKS

Striking a Balance

The secret of long-term weight loss does not lie in counting calories: it lies in striking a balance by making sure that the different types of food on your plate are there in the right proportions. You should get more of your calories from high-carbohydrate foods and fewer from fat.

The right balance

No diet in the world would tell you to eat as much as you like and still lose weight – if you find one that does, ignore it. There must be a few guidelines, but these do not need to be too harsh or extreme. A diet will not work if you cannot keep it up over the long term.

A high-carbohydrate and low-fat diet provides energy and nutrients without overloading on calories, but since very few foods are 100% carbohydrate, protein, or fat, you need to learn to recognize what different foods are made of, then mix and match them to create a diet that follows the guidelines below.

Eat unlimited

Choose fresh or frozen fruit and vegetables in preference to canned, and eat them raw or lightly cooked to preserve nutrients. Eat at least five types a day to ensure a healthy vitamin, mineral, and fiber intake.

Eat frequently

At least 50% of everything you eat should be

Eat sparingly

Eat in moderation

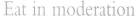
Eat frequently

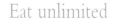
Eat unlimited

carbohydrates. If you view carbohydrates with a degree of suspicion, this might seem high. The high-protein/low-carbohydrate diet (see pages 30 – 31) of the Seventies convinced many of us that potatoes and pasta are fattening. Yet there are plenty of examples of people who maintain lean physiques on even higher proportions of carbohydrates: in the Far East, for instance, rice traditionally provides around 80% of calories. Obesity has only recently become a problem in Japan, and it is directly related to the introduction of a Western diet that is high in protein and fat and low in carbohydrates. Medical opinion stands firm: it is easier to store the fat you eat as body fat than it is to store carbohydrates as fat. To increase your carbohydrate intake, eat plenty of sugar-free breakfast cereals, bread, pasta, and rice (see pages 28 – 29). Whole-grain varieties are preferable because they contain more vitamins, minerals, and fiber.

Eat in moderation

Between 10 and 20% of your diet should be protein, which amounts to around two servings a day. The adult daily requirement for protein is probably lower than you think, and most of us eat more than enough protein without even trying. In developed nations, protein deficiency is virtually nonexistent. Although children and pregnant women need slightly more, an adult weighing 132lb (60kg) has a daily requirement of only 1½oz (45g). In theory, 7oz (200g) of shrimp would provide all the protein needed. In reality, the protein in your diet must come from a wide variety of foods to ensure a balance of essential amino acids (see pages 30 – 31). Protein is present in most foods. Meat and dairy products are high in protein, but since they can also be high in fat, choose lean meat, poultry without the skin, and low-fat cheese and milk. Dried beans, tofu, and fish are also good low-fat sources of protein.

Eat sparingly

Fat should make up no more than 30% of your diet. This means foods high in fat should, for the most part, be avoided since nearly everyone can afford to reduce the amount of fat they eat. But however desperately you want to lose weight, do not try to cut out fat completely; it is an essential part of a balanced diet. Fat is a component of most foods, so you probably eat much more than you realize. If you are used to a high-fat diet, you may initially miss the flavor, but tastebuds can be educated; cut down gradually on the fat you eat, and you may even find you don't like it anymore. Keep an eye on the type of fat you are eating; two-thirds of it should be unsaturated (see pages 32 – 33).

How to read food labels

The information on the back of a package of food is not there just to entertain you during breakfast; it is there to help you make informed decisions about what you eat. Most packaging carries a list of ingredients and a nutritional table. Learning how to make sense of labeling will allow you to see at a glance whether what you are eating is nutritionally sound.

How to get it right

Ingredients Listed according to amount, the ingredient that comes first is present in the largest quantity. Study a few food labels, and you may be surprised at what the food contains: vegetable oil can be high in the list of ingredients for cakes, cookies, and even breakfast cereals. Food manufacturers have been known to use misleading descriptions, so beware. Vegetable oil can often mean coconut oil: not exactly a vegetable and, unlike all other vegetables, it is high in saturated fat.

The nutritional table

This describes the nutritional quality of the product you are buying. It isn't required to list all the ingredients: you may notice entries such as "spices" or "natural flavors."

Calories The figure given tells you how many calories there are and usually specifies calories from fat. Food can be low-calorie yet still be mainly made up of refined sugar and fat.

Protein Shown only as a total amount, you need to look at the list of ingredients to determine if the protein comes from animal or vegetable sources. Protein is present to some degree in almost all food.

Carbohydrates These are usually divided into fiber and sugar, or refined and complex carbohydrates.

Alternatively, sugars can be listed under the general heading of "Carbohydrate," which makes it difficult to check the amount of refined sugar added. Sugar provides energy but is of little nutritional value.

Total fat content This is often followed by a figure showing how much of the total amount of fat is saturated. All fat is equally fattening, but unsaturated fat is a healthier choice. Beware: reduced-fat foods can contain up to 40% fat.

Additional information Some nutrition tables list elements that are known to have implications on health, such as sodium (a component of salt), vitamins and minerals, or fiber. The presence of fiber sometimes indicates that the carbohydrates are unrefined, although this isn't always the case.

Using common sense

When there is no nutritional table, you must use your own judgement to estimate the likely fat content. Remember the following hints:

Fat makes food greasy If your fingers are greasy after handling food, you can assume that it is high in fat. Sugary foods tends to make your fingers feel sticky.

Saturated fat tends to solidify At room temperature, saturated fats harden, which can be quite useful: when stews and soups are left to cool, the fat forms a crust over the top that can be easily removed, substantially lowering their fat content.

Fatty foods "melt down" Animal fats are hard when they come out of the refrigerator, but when heated they melt. The fat in sausages and burgers, for instance, melts when cooked and can be drained away or dabbed with a paper towel.

Cut down on processed foods Pies, cakes, cookies, and frozen dinners are often laden with hidden sugars and fats.

Seven-point Plan

Now that you know the facts about dieting, you can understand why weight loss does not – cannot – happen overnight. Losing weight is about eating sensibly in the long term, not about starving yourself. You need a strategy that you can stick to: a well-formulated plan rooted in fact and not in fiction.

1 Modify your diet by striking the right balance between the types of food you eat (see pages 38 – 39). This means cutting down on fat and increasing the amount of carbohydrates in your diet. The Good Food Guides (see pages 42 – 49) will help you do this.

2 Eat little and often. Convention dictates we eat three square meals a day, with a break of several hours between. We aren't designed to go so long without food, which is why the snack-food industry prospers. Rather than three big meals, eat three smaller meals and two high-carbohydrate, low-fat snacks.

3 Don't skip meals. It encourages your body to crave food and, if it becomes something of a "forbidden fruit," the desire to eat can be overwhelming, regardless of how hungry you really are. Eating sufficient carbohydrates in small, frequent meals, will reassure the body it will be fed regularly.

4 Cut down on alcohol. Sorry about this, but alcohol does contain a lot of calories that are very rarely put to good use. Although it may initially appear to perk you up, alcohol has a sedative effect and will make you much less inclined to use the energy those calories provide.

5 Drink more water. It does not make you fat, and few people drink enough. Neither tea nor coffee are particularly good for quenching thirst since they both contain caffeine, which is a diuretic and speeds up the rate of urine loss. Substitute bottled water, or try fruit or herbal teas. If you're not used to them, try several before you decide you don't like them; fruit flavors are less bitter than herbal teas.

6 The Total Fitness Plan (see pages 50 – 91) will help you get rid of excess body fat. Do it at least three, and preferably five, times a week. The strength training section (see pages 64 – 79) can on occasion be omitted, but never skip the aerobic section.

7 Persevere. Don't be tempted to fall for any of those dieting fantasies: starving yourself as punishment for one indulgence won't help. We all fall off the wagon sometimes, so don't hate yourself for it. One chocolate doesn't make or break a diet, but eating the whole box because you didn't have one when you wanted it probably will. Getting it nearly right each day is better than perfection once a week.

The Good Food Guides

The Good Food Guides are designed to steer you safely through the day by offering nutritious suggestions for breakfast, lunch, dinner and snacks. They are full of ideas for spicing up a high-carbohydrate, low-fat diet, but you don't have to follow them slavishly.

This is not a recipe book – there are no specific recipes for controling your weight and there are plenty of other books available that can tell you how to prepare delicious, low-fat meals. Neither is it a diet book, at least not in the traditional sense: it doesn't dictate a detailed weekly menu and then leave you to guess what to do when you reach the end of it. A diet will not work if it's repetitious and boring, or if you are forced to eat foods you do not particularly like. If it is going to be successful, an eating plan has to prepare you to make your own informed decisions about what to eat in the long term.

As long as you stay within the guidelines, you can adapt the suggestions that follow to suit your taste. Once you are armed with the information you need to balance your diet, it is easy to make the right choices.

The Good Breakfast Guide

Breakfast is probably the most important meal of the day. It is – literally – the breaking of the overnight fast. Although you have been sleeping, your body has been using energy to carry out repairs and to stay alive. Breakfast is your chance to refuel.

Research reveals two interesting facts about breakfast

1 People who skip breakfast are more likely to be overweight than those who regularly eat breakfast.

2 In tests, people who were given a high-carbohydrate breakfast voluntarily chose to eat less later in the day.

It is especially important to start the day with a high-carbohydrate meal. It will give you the energy you need to get to work and enhance your mental ability when you get there: research has shown that children who eat a high-carbohydrate breakfast do better in school tests than those who have a high-fat breakfast, like bacon and eggs. Try some of the followings ideas:

- Granola with low-fat yogurt and fruit
- Any high-fiber cereal without added sugar
- Dried fruit – apricots, figs, dates, and prunes
- Low-fat yogurt with puréed apples or peaches, flavored with cinnamon or nutmeg
- Oatmeal with blackberries or other soft fruit
- Whole-wheat toast or bagels with a low-sugar/ high-fruit jam – gradually cut out butter, or try to find a low-fat, unhydrogenated spread
- Freshly squeezed fruit juice – a good source of vitamin C, carbohydrates, and fluid
- English muffins with broiled pineapple or mango
- Blend together banana, melon, yogurt, and orange juice
- Broiled tomatoes on toasted soda bread
- Pancakes with sliced banana and low-fat yogurt
- Limit yourself to a single cup of tea or coffee with low-fat milk, or try herbal or fruit teas.

The Good Lunch Guide

Lunch is a meal that is often taken on the run. Very few of us have the time to sit down for a three-course feast. This isn't necessarily a bad thing; digesting large meals often makes you feel lethargic. It makes more sense to have a lighter lunch and a reasonably sized snack (see pages 48 – 49) on either side of it.

Plan ahead

If you know you are going to be away from home during the day without access to good, healthy food, it is a good idea to prepare your lunch in advance; fill a Thermos with soup, make a salad or sandwich, and take it with you.

Sandwiches
There are so many types of bread available now – ciabatta, focaccia, pita, naan, rye, and soda bread – that the sandwich is no longer a boring option. Choose whole-grain bread over refined white bread, because the fiber makes it more filling. Opt for sandwiches and rolls with more bread than filling. Fillings should be low in fat, so avoid regular mayonnaise, butter, margarine, fatty meat, or cheese. Good fillings include:
- Grilled chicken or turkey, with watercress and cucumber
- Low-fat cream cheese with mint and sliced fresh apricots or peaches
- Low-fat hummus, grated carrot, and chopped fresh cilantro or mint
- Mashed banana with cottage cheese
- Low-fat mozzarella, sliced tomato, and fresh basil
- Low-fat vegetable pâté.

Baked potatoes
Easy to cook, baked potatoes provide plenty of long-term energy. They are high in fiber and contain only a trace of fat. Baked sweet potatoes are a good alternative. Fillings should be low in fat, so avoid butter and cheese, and choose from the following:
- Tuna, corn, red kidney beans, celery, scallions, and low-fat mayonnaise

■ Baked beans spiced with Tabasco, Worcestershire sauce, or chili sauce, and chopped tomato
■ Broiled tomatoes, fresh herbs, and seasoning
■ Cottage cheese with a spoonful of pesto
■ Lightly sautéed mushrooms with garlic, chopped chives, and a spoonful of plain yogurt
■ Salsa: chopped tomatoes, peppers, chili, fresh herbs, and lemon juice.

Pasta Naturally low in fat and high in carbohydrates, pasta is an excellent source of energy, but choose your sauce carefully; pasta is easily transformed into a high-fat dish by adding a cheese- or cream-based sauce. Try the following options:
■ A tomato-based sauce, or finely sliced zucchini or other raw vegetables, tossed with pasta and a small spoonful of olive oil and freshly ground black pepper
■ Pesto sauce: although it contains quite a lot of oil, you need to use so little that it is not a bad choice
■ Steamed broccoli and chopped fresh chili sautéed in a little olive oil.

Rice Substantial and filling, rice can make a complete meal in itself when it is combined with a few other ingredients. Brown rice has more fiber, vitamins, and minerals than white rice. Couscous or bulghar wheat are equally good. Try some of the following recipe ideas:
■ Add raisins and a few almonds to saffron rice
■ Stir blanched spinach leaves and diced broiled chicken into rice that has been cooked in a stock made with garlic, cumin seeds, and turmeric
■ Tuna, chopped fresh chilies, tomatoes, and fresh basil stirred into cooked rice.

Soup Serve with bread, preferably whole-grain. Try the following combinations:
■ Cook sliced onion in a little oil, add a selection of vegetables – carrots, celery, zucchini, peppers, peas, tomatoes, potatoes – add vegetable stock, season, cook until all the vegetables are tender, and blend to make a creamy, filling soup
■ Add canned beans – chick peas, cannellini, lentils – as a nutritious supplement to the above
■ Add sliced scallions and fresh ginger to vegetable stock, pour over cooked egg noodles, and sprinkle with cilantro. Tofu adds a low-fat source of protein to this soup.

Salad Although salads are a good source of vitamins and cancer-preventing nutrients, you should avoid adding fatty meat, fried croutons, and avocado, which (for a fruit) is surprisingly high in fat. Similarly, salads are easily turned from a nutritious lunch into a source of fat by adding ladles of dressing. The following are low-fat combinations:
■ Add high-carbohydrate foods such as corn, kidney beans, lentils, chick peas, rice, or pasta to chopped peppers, mushrooms, onion, celery, and fresh herbs
■ Watercress or fennel mixed with sliced oranges
■ Toasted sunflower seeds or sesame seeds sprinkled over a mixed-leaf salad dressed with balsamic vinegar or lemon juice
■ Grated carrots combined with grated fresh ginger, chives, lime juice, and a few drops of sesame oil.

Soup can make a nutritious and substantial lunch. Serve with plenty of whole-grain bread

The Good Dinner Guide

If you are cooking at home, it is easy to ensure that the food you eat is low in fat and high in carbohydrates. When you eat out, stick to the same criteria – avoid foods that are obviously fatty, like cream- or cheese-based sauces, or anything fried.

Meal planning

Base meals around carbohydrate foods, like pasta, rice, and potatoes, rather than the traditional approach, where meat is the central feature. Serve the following dishes with plenty of vegetables, preferably broiled, steamed, or roasted, or a large tossed salad:

Pasta Serve pasta with tomato or vegetable sauces, instead of high-fat meat or cream sauces. For a simple fresh tomato sauce, lightly brush halved tomatoes with a little olive oil and roast in an oven for 30 minutes. In a food processor, blend the roasted tomatoes with chopped chili, garlic, and basil leaves, and serve.

Rice Although available in many guises, brown rice is the most nutritious, packed with vitamins, minerals, and fiber. Cook brown rice in a vegetable stock with sliced dried apricots. Fry sliced onion in a little olive oil, and add ground cumin, coriander, and chili powder. Roast cubes of pumpkin or sweet potato that have been lightly brushed with oil, and mix with the rice and spices.

Fish Filets or steaks of fish can be given an Oriental flavor: blend together fresh ginger, soy sauce, lemon juice, scallions, and five-spice powder in a food processor until they form a thick paste. Spread over fish and broil.

Meat Choose lean cuts of meat, and trim off any obvious fat before cooking. Use a cooking method that allows the fat to drain away – broiling or roasting, rather than frying. Dab meat with paper towels to soak up any excess fat after cooking. Marinades add flavor to meat without adding extra fat. For a Moroccan-inspired marinade combine lemon juice with chili powder, cumin, paprika, and a splash of olive oil. Marinate cubed lean lamb, chicken, or fish for at least one hour before broiling.

Poultry Eat more broiled chicken or turkey. Much of the fat in poultry lies under and in the skin. Remove the skin before cooking to prevent the fat from seeping into the flesh as it cooks. The marinades for meat or fish are equally good with poultry.

Pizza This can make a well-balanced meal, especially when the crust is thick or deep-

pan. It is the pizza topping that can be a problem. Avoid meat, keep high-fat cheese to a minimum, and choose vegetable-based toppings instead. Top a pizza base with a fresh tomato sauce or a thin layer of pesto sauce or olive paste, and add thinly sliced mushrooms, peppers, tomatoes, and garlic. Sprinkle with fresh or dried oregano or fresh basil. Drizzle with olive oil, if desired, and bake in the oven until crisp and golden.

Vegetables Most of us do not eat enough vegetables, yet they contain vital vitamins and minerals, and they are very low in fat. Allow vegetables to form the central part of a meal: stuff peppers or eggplants with a mix of onions, peppers, zucchini, and tomatoes cooked in a little olive oil. Bake in the oven for one hour and serve with rice. For variety, add tuna, corn, or black or pinto beans. Puréed vegetables also make simple and nutritious sauces and soups.

Potatoes To replace fries, cut potatoes into wedge shapes, lay on a baking tray, season, and drizzle with a little olive oil. Bake in a oven for one hour, until golden. Alternatively, thinly slice potatoes and combine with sliced onion, tomato, fresh rosemary, and garlic in a baking dish. Pour in some vegetable stock, cover with foil, and bake in the oven for one hour.

Room for dessert

If you eat a main course that is high in carbohydrates, you will probably find that you do not have room for dessert. However, if you are still hungry, here are some healthy options:
- Fresh fruit – melon, kiwi fruit, grapes
- Low-fat yogurt mixed with fruit and sunflower seeds, or sweetened with a little honey
- Baked apple stuffed with raisins, dates, or dried apricots and a little honey
- Low-fat rice pudding, sprinkled with grated nutmeg
- Puréed mango or pineapple mixed into plain yogurt or low-fat fromage frais
- For a simple fruit sauce, combine frozen raspberries and strawberries in a blender (add a little sugar if the fruit is very tart). Pass the purée through a sieve to remove the seeds, and serve warm or cold with a low-fat yogurt or a fruit sorbet
- Stewed dried fruit – figs, dates, apricots, apples, raisins, peaches, and pears

Be imaginative in your use of vegetables – they can form the central part of a meal

The Good Snack Guide

The point of snacking is to bridge the gap between main meals and keep blood sugar levels constant. When blood sugar fluctuates, so does energy. To avoid this, you should snack on foods where the calories come from carbohydrates, not from fat.

Healthy snacks

Many snack foods are very high in fat. We all underestimate how much we eat, and it is easy to overlook the odd handful of peanuts now and then, but that bit can add considerably to the total amount of fat you eat. To avoid temptation, create a "safe" environment in your home or workplace by surrounding yourself with plenty of low-fat foods to snack on. If you feel an irresistible craving for something indulgent, it's better to go for an unbuttered scone or muffin rather than a packet of peanuts.

Fruit
The perfect snack food, fruit even comes pre-wrapped. Where fruit is concerned, there are no restrictions; no fruit (except avocado) is more "fattening" than any other. Fruit contains practically no fat at all. It consists mainly of carbohydrates and water – at least 50% – and is high in vitamins too.

Dried fruit
A compact source of healthy sugar. Dried fruit retains its carbohydrates and fiber, but vitamins are lost with the water. Dried apricots, raisins, and prunes are high in iron.

Raw vegetables
Often overlooked as a snack food, probably because most vegetables need some preparation before they are eaten. In fact, if washed, many vegetables can be eaten raw. They are a good source of carbohydrates, and contain plenty of vitamins, minerals, and fiber.

Pita bread Low-fat hummus, salad, or broiled vegetables mixed with a little pesto sauce or olive tapenade make delicious fillings for pita bread.

English muffins and scones These are both good sources of carbohydrates, which are easily spoiled by the addition of butter and cream cheese. Muffins and scones have a natural sweetness, so try them on their own, or top them with soft fruit, such as strawberries, raspberries, or blueberries and a spoonful of low-fat yogurt. If you really cannot give up spreads, switch to a low-fat type. These contain about half the fat of butter, but look for one that is unhydrogenated (see page 33), as it is much better for your health.

Bagels Versatile and convenient, bagels are available in many different kinds. Onion and pumpernickel bagels can be eaten with a thin layer of low-fat cream cheese, cottage cheese with chives or scallions, or low-fat vegetable pâté. Sweet bagels, such as cinnamon and raisin, do not need much in the way of topping and are perfect toasted with sliced banana or low-sugar, high-fruit jam.

Rice cakes Nibble plain, or top with absolutely anything – vegetables, fresh fruit, jam, or cottage cheese.

Pretzels An excellent source of carbohydrates, but avoid those that are heavily coated in salt.

Popcorn A healthy snack, as long as the popcorn is not coated with oil, butter, or salt. Try making popcorn yourself and flavoring it with paprika, soy sauce, Tabasco, or, for a sweet alternative, cinnamon or nutmeg. Avoid the ready-made, caramel-coated variety – the coating is pure refined sugar.

Low-fat cookies Lower in fat than normal cookies, but check the label as many low-fat cookies are loaded with refined sugar to compensate for the lack of taste. They are often just as high in calories – they just come from a different source.

Sandwiches An excellent high-carbohydrate snack, as long as the filling is low in fat. For filling ideas see pages 44 – 45.

Breadsticks Can be eaten on their own, or can be dipped into low-fat hummus or tzatziki.

Yogurt All yogurt is made with milk, but this is often where the similarity ends. It can be made with whole or skim milk and sometimes has added sugar, cream, fruit, or other flavorings. Similarly, the fat content can vary from 0.01oz (0.2g) per 3.5oz (100g) in low-fat yogurt to 0.3oz (9g) per 3.5oz (100g) in whole-milk yogurt. Plain yogurt can be flavored with fresh or dried fruit, fruit purée, or cinnamon, or can be used as a low-fat salad dressing. Low-fat creme fraiche is now becoming more available.

Sandwiches and rolls make an excellent high-carbohydrate snack

49

Total Fitness Plan

I am no stranger to exercise – I have been dancing for most of my life – but the first time I decided to exercise for *fitness*, I felt as if I were crashing a private party.

Fitness has become a bit exclusive: you probably think you need to buy the right gear, join a gym, or hire a personal trainer if you're serious about getting fit.

In fact, you don't need to do any of these things. All you need to get fit is a good pair of shoes, the right advice, and a healthy dose of determination. It will all feel a bit strange at first, but bear in mind an old Norwegian saying: "The mile across the doorstep is the longest."

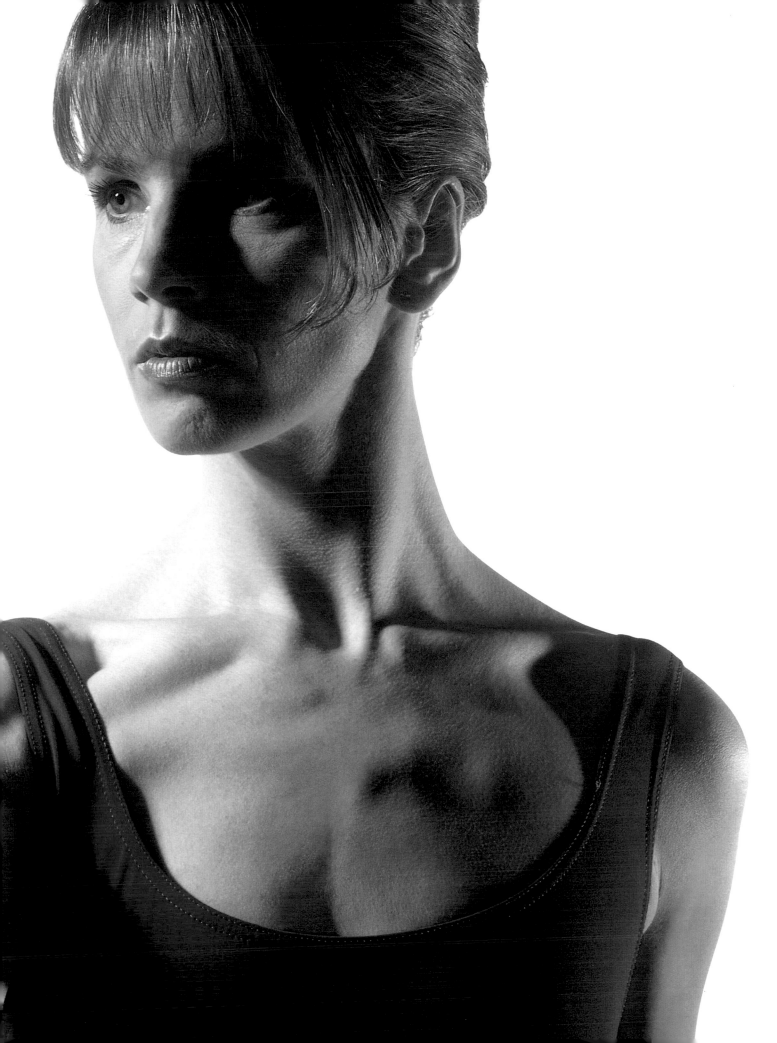

Getting the Right Gear

There are no hard and fast rules about what to wear when you exercise, unless you intend to take up competitive athletics. In some ways, the most important thing is to feel comfortable. However, since all physical exercise involves sweating – you're going to get wet – some clothes are more suitable than others.

Keeping warm, staying cool

The evaporation of sweat is the body's cooling mechanism. In windy weather, when evaporation is rapid, you risk cooling down too much. The trick is to wear "breathable" clothing that allows sweat to evaporate yet keeps you warm throughout your workout (see side bar). Always wear socks: the Achilles' tendon is never very warm, and a cold tendon is at risk of injury. There is also a practical concern – without socks, sweat quickly rots shoes.

WARM WEATHER

Shorts or warm-up pants and a loose T-shirt.

This is the only weather when shorts are suitable: sweating limbs are best covered up. In intense sunshine, use a sweat-resistant sunscreen to avoid getting burned.

COOL WEATHER

Warm-up pants and a top of moisture-transporting fabric, such as polypropylene.

You can add a sweatshirt and (if it's windy) a breathable windbreaker.

COLD WEATHER

Moisture-transporting fabric on the legs and upper body.

You can cover this with warm-up pants and a thin wool layer, such as an old sweater. You may need a breathable windbreaker, gloves, and even a woolen hat.

Shoes

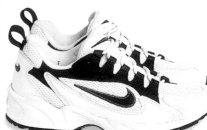

To avoid the risk of injury, you should always wear good shoes: this may be the one expense necessary before you can begin. Appropriate shoes are especially important if you plan on jogging

Helmet

Never cycle without this – both a helmet and visible clothing are essential

Bike

For general training, choose a "hybrid" bike. Mountain bikes are really for serious off-road cycling, although "slick" tires will make them smoother for road use

A firm footing

If you're not used to physical activity, exercise will put an unfamiliar strain on your joints, muscles, and tendons. It is vital that you give them as much support as possible by wearing the best shoes that you can afford; don't be tempted to go out in your cheap old sneakers. Hang on to them, though; they can provide valuable information for later.

Go to an athletic store and ask for a shoe designed to support your particular type of feet. Take your old shoes with you – they will provide valuable clues as to the sort of shoes you should buy as a replacement.

There are basically three types of feet (see right): flat, "pronating" feet that roll inward, high-arched "supinating" feet that roll outward, and "neutral" feet that are more or less straight. When the feet roll either way, the shoes need to compensate. Pronating feet need "straight-lasted" shoes with good arch- and medial support. Supinating feet need shoes with good arch- and lateral support, and especially good shock

absorbency, since these feet can be rather rigid. All shoes should be snug, but not tight, and have good shock absorbency. Unless you intend to run only on dry pavements, avoid smooth-soled shoes, which will be slippery in wet or muddy conditions. Try several pairs before you decide – don't just go for the ones with the nicest colors. Shoes should be chosen with the feet, not the eyes.

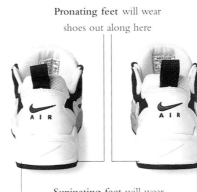

Pronating feet will wear shoes out along here

Supinating feet will wear shoes out along here

WIND CHILL

However warm the temperature, wind speed can have a dramatic effect on how warm you feel. This is known as the wind-chill factor. Cyclists should pay particular attention to the wind chill, since cycling into the wind increases its cooling effect.

Chin-up bar

Mount a bar just beyond your maximum reach, so it can be used for the hanging stretch. Always check it is secure before use

Elastic band

There are several types available – choose an inexpensive, basic version made of good-quality rubber

Bike stand

If you already own a bicycle, this is a cheaper option than buying a stationary exercise bike

Heart-rate monitor

An easy way of checking that you are exercising at the right intensity. Choose a basic, inexpensive model

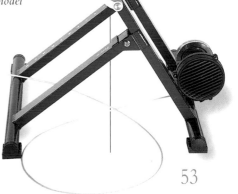

When To Exercise

It doesn't matter what time of the day you exercise. Although some experts claim that a morning work-out raises the metabolic rate and keeps it elevated for the rest of the day, others have found no evidence of any "afterburning" effect. Ultimately it comes down to practicalities. You need to find a space in the day that suits you.

Eating and exercise

Fitting exercise around meals requires a little planning. You obviously don't want to work out feeling hungry, nor do you want to feel bloated. Finding a balance between the two is a question of timing. If you are exercising primarily to burn fat, it is especially important not to eat just beforehand. In response to food, the pancreas releases the hormone insulin, which *temporarily* prevents fat from being used as a source of energy.

A question of timing

Digesting a large meal takes several hours, and during this time you won't feel very energetic. There are two reasons for this: First, blood is diverted to the stomach to digest the food, so there is less blood available to carry oxygen to the muscles. Second, the pancreas releases insulin, and this may make you feel lethargic. The brain requires a constant level of sugar in the blood, and insulin helps to regulate this. When food is digested, the sugar it contains is absorbed into the bloodstream, and the blood sugar level goes up. To counteract this, insulin is released to "push" this sugar into the muscles and liver. The consequent drop in blood sugar often brings a temporary feeling of tiredness. Refined sugars, which release their energy in one great surge, cause the insulin to overcompensate, which can lead to bouts of dizziness.

You should allow at least two hours between eating and exercise so that you aren't affected by any dips in energy levels. If you've eaten sufficient carbohydrates, you'll have plenty of stored energy available. Work-outs lasting less than 90 minutes rely entirely on stored fuel; it's only when you exercise for longer than this that food eaten *immediately* before (or during) exercise starts to provide energy.

If you choose to work out first thing in the morning, it can be difficult to fit in breakfast beforehand. Have some fruit or a glass of fruit juice half an hour before you start; this will be enough to get you going. Be sure to eat breakfast afterward.

Energy drinks

Marketers are a bit unscrupulous when they use the word "energy," failing to mention that "low *calorie*" means low *energy*, or that "energy" drinks provide energy because they are high in calories.

If you are ill, energy drinks can be very useful, and if you're running a marathon, they can be a lifeline. But if your main objective is to burn fat, energy drinks may not be a good idea, since the sugar content causes the pancreas to produce insulin. While there is a high level of insulin in the blood, fat cannot be used for energy. If you feel listless or lethargic, take a look at your diet and your lifestyle. Don't imagine you can open a bottle and instantly solve the problem.

CAUTION

When NOT To Exercise:

Consistency is one of the most important factors in an exercise program to burn fat, but there are some occasions when you should take a rain check:

If you feel at all unwell.

If you have a temperature.

If you have any aches and pains above and beyond the stiffness associated with increased activity.

You must stop immediately if you feel any pain, dizziness, or faintness during exercise.

In any of these circumstances, see your doctor before you resume the exercise program.

The Pre-Exercise Plan

Unless you're very fit, it's not a good idea to launch into exercise without a little preparation. Most important, leaping directly from the sofa to a 30-minute workout puts you at risk of injury. Even if you escape this, you would ache so much from the unfamiliar activity that you would probably give up on day two.

The three starting levels

Depending on your general fitness, your body takes at least two weeks to adjust to any increase in activity. During this time, the overriding concern is injury prevention. Don't worry that you're not burning fat: it is more important to strengthen your muscles, tendons, and ligaments so that you can eventually follow the Total Fitness Plan without interruption from injury. Be sure to complete level three before you move on to the fitness plan.

Where to begin

Every novice exerciser starts from a different level – be honest with yourself, and choose the one on the right that best describes your general fitness. Finish each fitness session with a light stretch (see pages 58–59). When you have completed one level, move on to the next. Once you have completed level three, you are ready to start the Total Fitness Plan.

It's also a good idea to start increasing your general level of activity – by choosing a more active option, you give a much-needed boost to your metabolism. Any of the following can be easily built into your daily routine:

■ Cycle or walk to work.
■ If you live too far to walk all the way, park farther from the office, and walk the last couple of miles.
■ Get off the bus or subway a few stops early. You might also save money!
■ Walk up stairs instead of taking the elevator or the escalator.
■ Don't use the car for short trips – walk or cycle instead.

LEVEL 1
YEARS OF NEGLECT

Unable to walk up a flight of stairs without stopping.
Two weeks of the following:

■ *45 seconds of slow walking*
■ *15 seconds of fast walking*
■ *Start this cycle with 5 minutes daily, adding 1 minute every second day. Follow this with the light stretch.*

LEVEL 2
UNFIT

Out of breath after climbing a flight of stairs.
Two weeks of the following:

■ *1 minute of slow walking*
■ *1 minute of fast walking*
■ *Start this cycle with 10 minutes daily, adding 1 minute every second day. Follow this with the light stretch.*

LEVEL 3
FAIRLY FIT

No restrictions in day-to-day activity.
Two weeks of the following:

■ *1 minute of slow walking*
■ *30 seconds of easy jogging*
■ *Start this cycle with 10 minutes daily, adding 1 minute every second day. Follow this with the light stretch.*

The Fitness Plan

TOTAL FITNESS PLAN

It consists of six parts, the "six pack" of fitness:

■

WARMUP

■

LIGHT STRETCH

■

THE AEROBIC ELEMENT

■

COOL-DOWN

■

STRENGTH TRAINING

■

FULL STRETCH

Easy to follow, safe, and effective, the Total Fitness Plan is designed to allow you to make your own decisions about the type of exercise you want to do and where you'd like to do it. The only real expense is the cost of a good pair of shoes, although if you want to join a gym, there is nothing to stop you: running on a treadmill is just as effective as running outdoors, except the scenery isn't quite as good.

A well-equipped gym offers the option of machines for strength training, but I have become quite adept at finding very effective substitutes. Your own body weight provides tailor-made resistance, and working against it is an excellent way to build strength. You will need an elastic exercise band, but these are not expensive, and you can even use an old bicycle inner tube. A sturdy tree branch can double as a chin-up bar, and a park bench is useful for stretching as well as for chair dips and abdominal and hamstring exercises.

The Total Fitness Plan works equally well for weight loss and weight maintenance. You need to do it at least three, and preferably five, times a week. The more you do it, the more fat you will burn, but don't forget that the body needs an occasional day off. It contains everything you need to lose body fat, maintain and build muscle strength, improve posture, and benefit health. It is a fitness package to last a lifetime.

Warm Up

Don't be tempted to skimp on your warmup. It's an essential part of your workout. Until you're properly warm, your muscles and tendons are much less pliable and therefore less able to cope with the demands of exercise. Exercising without a good warmup significantly increases your risk of injury.

Increasing the temperature

Most materials are more flexible when they are warm. Elements as diverse as metal and wax can be molded once their temperature is increased, and human tissue is no different. You often see people trying to "stretch" before they start their workout, but until the connective tissue in the muscles is warm, stretching is much less effective.

Increasing the pace

Warming up is not only about the muscles in your arms and legs. The heart is also a muscle. A good warmup should raise the heart rate gradually to the level where it can pump enough oxygenated blood around the body to meet the increasing demand from the working muscles. Until then, exercise has to be anaerobic (without oxygen), and the build-up of lactic acid will make your legs feel tired (see page 20). Don't let this put you off: the muscles will very soon be supplied with oxygen, and the lactic acid will be recycled. Remember, the beginning is always the hardest part.

The most efficient way to warm up is also the simplest: start the activity you intend to do at a very gentle level, and increase the pace over about 5 to 10 minutes. For example, if you are going to run, begin by walking for a few minutes, then step up the pace until it becomes a fast walk/easy jog. You can alternate between two minutes of walking and two of jogging. If you are cycling, start in the easiest gear, and shift up one or two gears every minute. Some types of aerobic exercise may not adapt so easily to become a warmup, but you can safely substitute the walking/jogging formula instead.

Warming up gently introduces the muscles to the movements they are about to do, and because coordination improves after a few minutes of practice, an appropriate warmup also reduces the risk of injury.

A warmup that uses large muscle groups, such as the thighs and hamstrings, will obviously be more effective, since it works the heart harder: large muscles need more oxygen than smaller ones. An effective warmup should bring on a light sweat and leave you breathing hard, but not gasping for breath. If you are already warm, exercise will be effective from the outset.

Light Stretch

Now that you're warm, you should gently stretch before going on to your aerobic exercise. Stretching gradually increases muscle length and flexibility, and long, flexible muscles are less prone to injury. Stretching also acts as a "check point": use it to test that everything is working smoothly before you continue with the next section.

LIGHT STRETCH

See pages 80–91 for detailed information on the stretches. For now, they need only be done once on each side:

■

INNER THIGH STRETCH

■

HIP FLEXOR STRETCH

■

FRONT THIGH STRETCH

■

HAMSTRINGS STRETCH

■

UPPER AND LOWER CALF STRETCH

Easy does it

You don't need to push too hard at this point – the full stretch will come later. Choose a suitable spot, with something (such as a bench) to hold on to, and don't pause for too long between the stretches. The whole thing should take no more than a couple of minutes – you don't want to lose the effect of your warmup.

The stretches

All the stretches in the Total Fitness Plan have been chosen because they stretch predominantly muscles that span two joints. They focus mostly on the muscles that attach to the pelvis and spine, as good mobility in this area is important in preventing lower-back pain.

Without muscles we would be completely immobile. Joints are made to move only by shortening the muscles that cross them. Any repetitive action (the definition of exercise) involves contracting the muscles over and over again, which can make them become tight. Stretching after exercise counteracts this, gently elongating the muscles while they are still warm. When the two-joint muscles are tight and shortened they can pull unevenly on the joints, leading to problems.

Stretching also serves as an opportunity to check that all the different parts of your body are in working order. Any increase in the amount of activity you do will inevitably leave the muscles feeling a little stiff and tired the next day; it is the recovery from stiffness that makes the muscles stronger. If you have any twinges above and beyond this, you should not continue to exercise.

In case of injury

Any fitness plan should put safety first, and you should not be at any risk while doing it. However, accidents do happen, and overenthusiasm – attempting to run before you can walk – can also put a strain on muscles, tendons, and ligaments, especially if they are not used to exercise. If you are unfortunate enough to injure yourself, don't try to "run it off." You must stop exercising immediately and remember one word: ICE.

I ce, if available, should be applied immediately and firmly to the injury. Use a wet cloth between the ice and bare skin to prevent ice "burn."

C ompression should always be used to prevent swelling. Tie a scarf, T-shirt, or anything else you can lay your hands on firmly around the injury.

E levate the injury above the level of the heart to further reduce the swelling that may occur. Discontinue exercise, and seek medical advice as soon as possible.

Increasing mobility

Over a period of time, stretching can actually lengthen the muscles, and it is through years of appropriate stretching that dancers and gymnasts achieve such extraordinary mobility.

Stretching should be done only when you are warm; cold muscles are much less elastic, and forcing them puts you at risk of injury. As part of your warmup, you need only do the stretches once on each side, since you are simply preparing your body for the aerobic exercise that will follow. To really feel the benefit, it is important to do them correctly and in the right order. Don't worry if it all sounds and feels rather strange in the beginning. You will very soon be your own expert.

"Focus on the muscles you are stretching, and feel them elongate as you hold the position."

Aerobic Exercise

The aerobic element is the part of your workout designed to burn fat. To achieve this effectively, you need to keep it up for at least 20 minutes at 60 – 70% of your heart's maximum capacity. Only then, when exercise is of the right intensity and duration, will the energy you use come from body fat.

Starting out

When you begin, you may find that brisk walking is enough to raise the heart rate to 60 – 70% of its capacity, especially if you are not used to exercise. As you get fitter, your heart, like the rest of your muscles, will become stronger, and you will need to increase the pace to push your heart rate to the right level.

Staying in the target zone

Because exercise needs to be of the right intensity to burn fat, it is important to work out your personal target zone before you start (see pages 22 – 23) and to keep within it. At first, you need to take your pulse at regular intervals to check that your heart is working at the right level. After a while, you will begin to recognize this level, using pace and breathing as indicators, and you won't need to test it quite so often. If you want to be really sure that you are within your target zone, you can buy a heart-rate monitor (see page 53).

A defining characteristic of aerobic exercise is that it can be sustained for long periods of time. If you can't keep going, it's probably because you've pushed your heart rate too high. Slow down to a walking pace, and gradually speed up again when it has returned to the target level. To burn a significant amount of fat you must keep going for at least 20 minutes.

If at first you find it difficult to train at a consistent pace for 20 – 30 minutes, try interval training (see tint box, below). Alternating between walking and jogging is the easiest form of interval training, and you can use the same principle for any type of activity. This type of training is often more enjoyable and can also be gentler on the joints than keeping a steady pace.

INTERVAL TRAINING

- *Once you have warmed up, jog until your heart rate reaches 70% of your maximum capacity (see pages 22 – 23).*
- *Slow down the pace to a walk until the heart rate drops to 60% of its maximum.*
- *Step up the pace until the heart rate reaches 70% again.*
- *Continue to alternate between the two for the duration of your workout.*

Choosing your exercise

There are several types of aerobic exercise, and you can choose whichever you like. Your heart doesn't know which type of exercise you are doing; it will register only the fact that your muscles require more oxygen. The "ideal" exercise for burning fat is the one that suits you best, although varying the activity from time to time will reduce the risk of overusing specific joints.

Brisk walking Probably the perfect exercise when you first start out, especially if you're very overweight. It's safe, familiar, low in impact, and easy to keep up.

Cross-country skiing If you have access to snow, this is an excellent form of exercise. Cross-country skiers are regularly shown to have the highest levels of fitness of all athletes and relatively low levels of body fat. Cross-country skiing uses all the major muscle groups in the arms and legs, and it is very low in impact. Many gyms have exercise machines that simulate cross-country skiing.

Cycling A good alternative to jogging. When cycling, the body weight is supported, so it's gentler on the joints. It does require some equipment – a helmet and visible clothing – but lots of people already own a bike. You do need to be mindful of the wind-chill factor. In bad weather, you can cycle indoors with the aid of a bike stand, which converts your bicycle into a stationary exercise bike (see page 53). These are quite inexpensive and can be bought at a good bike shop.

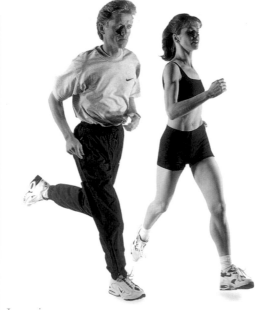

Jogging This is arguably the ultimate aerobic exercise, because it requires no equipment (other than a good pair of shoes) and works many of the large muscle groups. However, it probably isn't appropriate for absolute beginners, and it does increase the impact on the joints.

Mini trampoline Jogging can be done indoors, on the spot, with the help of a mini trampoline. This is very useful when it's raining and is very gentle on the joints. You can do any aerobic workout on a mini trampoline, and they are especially useful if you prefer to exercise to music.

Rowing The obvious downside to rowing is that you need either a boat or a rowing machine to do it. If you have access to either, it's a great form of exercise: it works the large muscle groups in both the upper and lower body. Since you do it sitting down, it is a non-impact activity. You need to take it easy at the beginning: it can be hard on the lower back.

Running in water This is much harder than it sounds – the effort of moving against the water's resistance makes it a very effective workout for the heart. Because you are more or less weightless, it's a good choice if you have any joint problems.

Swimming A non-weightbearing, nonimpact exercise that works all the major muscle groups against the resistance of the water. The only drawback may be that the cool water keeps the body temperature down, making it less effective in burning fat. It also requires access to a pool or suitable open water.

Exercise your imagination

Depending on the type you choose, aerobic exercise may or may not be all-weather. It is perfectly possible to run or cycle when it's raining, but if you don't like the idea of getting wet, you can (with a little imagination) adapt most aerobic exercise to be done indoors.

If it's possible, try to find a way to incorporate aerobic exercise into your existing daily routine. This isn't as hard as it sounds, and there are several ways in which it can be included (see page 55). One in three households, for instance, owns a bicycle, yet only one in three of those bicycles is ever used. If you have one hidden away, get it out and put it to good use. I would imagine that if everyone who lives within striking distance cycled to work instead of using the car, obesity, road congestion, and pollution could be cut in half at a single stroke.

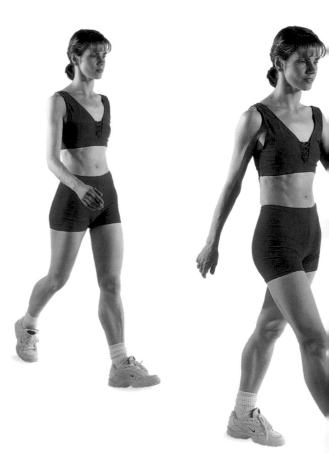

5-minute Cool-down

Like the warmup, the cool-down is a part of the Total Fitness Plan that you may be tempted to skip. Don't: it is as important as the warmup. Just as you raised your heart rate to the target level before you began, you must now bring it down again.

A proper cool-down will lower body temperature and help guard against any aches and pains.

Easing the pace

To cool down, you simply reverse your warmup. Gradually slow down the pace until your heart rate returns to normal. Whichever type of exercise you have been doing, you can use jogging as a cool-down: start out at a moderate pace, and slow to a walk over five minutes.

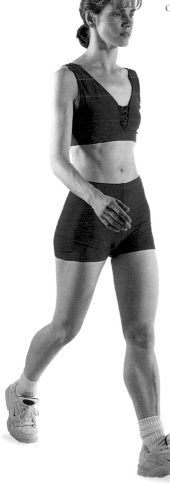

Strength Training

STRENGTH TRAINING

Follow the order in
which the exercises
are listed

■

ABDOMINALS
BACK EXTENSIONS

■

CHAIR DIPS
HAMSTRINGS

■

BICEPS
ARABESQUE

■

INNER THIGH
DELTOID

Strength training helps weight control by maintaining, and even increasing, muscle mass, which keeps the metabolic rate high. It also improves posture and reduces the risk of injury in daily physical tasks. The strength training will not burn fat in itself, which is why it is the only part of the Total Fitness Plan that can, on occasion, be omitted.

The exercises that follow are paired so that you can work one set of muscles while another set recovers, and you should do them in the order in which they appear. Start with the first of each pair given: focus on the muscles you are working, and do the exercise until the muscles are too tired to continue it correctly. Switch to the second exercise of the pair and follow the same procedure. You may want to repeat both exercises before moving on.

It is more important to do the exercises correctly than to aim for a specific number of repetitions (completed movements) but an amount you can work toward is suggested for each exercise, and you should eventually try to repeat each pair three times. The length of time it takes to achieve this will vary enormously from person to person. As a rough guide, it should take about three months to double the number of repetitions you can do. Don't worry if it takes longer: quality is more important than quantity.

Abdominals

The abdominals are a very important muscle group: strong abdominals support the spine. They also help to keep the stomach flat. Unless the abdominals are exercised with the hips and knees bent and supported, the psoas muscles do most of the work and the lower back is put under strain.

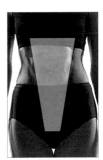

THE ABDOMINALS criss-cross the abdomen, with their main attachments at the lower ribs, breast bone, and pelvis.

1 *Lie on your back, with your calves resting on the seat of a chair, and your knees and hips supported at a 90° angle. Gently cup your hands around the back of your neck.*

Do not hook the feet in place

Keep the hips and knees bent at a 90° angle

2 *Contract your stomach muscles and raise your head and shoulders slightly off the ground.*

Do not pull the head forward with the hands

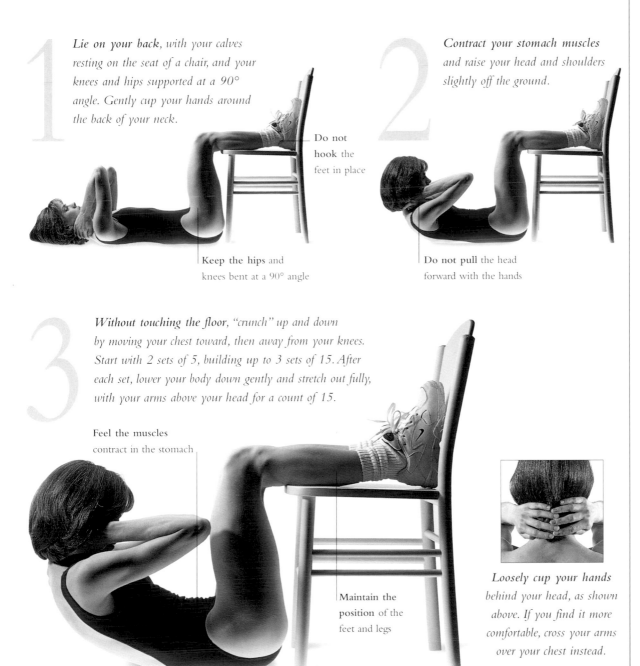

3 *Without touching the floor, "crunch" up and down by moving your chest toward, then away from your knees. Start with 2 sets of 5, building up to 3 sets of 15. After each set, lower your body down gently and stretch out fully, with your arms above your head for a count of 15.*

Feel the muscles contract in the stomach

Maintain the position of the feet and legs

Loosely cup your hands behind your head, as shown above. If you find it more comfortable, cross your arms over your chest instead.

CAUTION

Do not pull the head forward.

Do not hook the feet in place.

Do not twist the spine to target the "oblique" muscles. It can be dangerous, and this exercise works them sufficiently.

Back Extensions

This exercise targets most of the muscles in the back, especially the erector spinae muscles, which run prominently down both sides of the spine. Back extensions are important because they balance the strength of the abdominals and improve posture. If either the back or abdominal muscle groups are weak, there is a risk of lower back pain and injury.

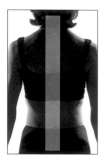

THE ERECTOR SPINAE MUSCLES are attached to each vertebra down the spine from the base of the skull to the pelvis.

1 *Lie face down, flat on the floor, with your arms stretched straight out above your head.*

2 *First tighten your buttock muscles, then lift your arms and legs steadily, so that your nose and knees are just off the ground. Hold this position for a count of 3, then gently lower your body. Relax for a count of 3, then repeat. Start with 2 sets of 3 lifts, building up to 3 sets of 10 lifts.*

CAUTION

Always tighten the buttocks before commencing step 2, to protect the lower back.

Do not lift the back or the legs too high off the ground.

Lift both arms and legs at a steady rate

Do not raise the head above the arms

The upper body lifts until the nose is just off the ground

"Back extensions

will help give you a dancer's

strength in your back."

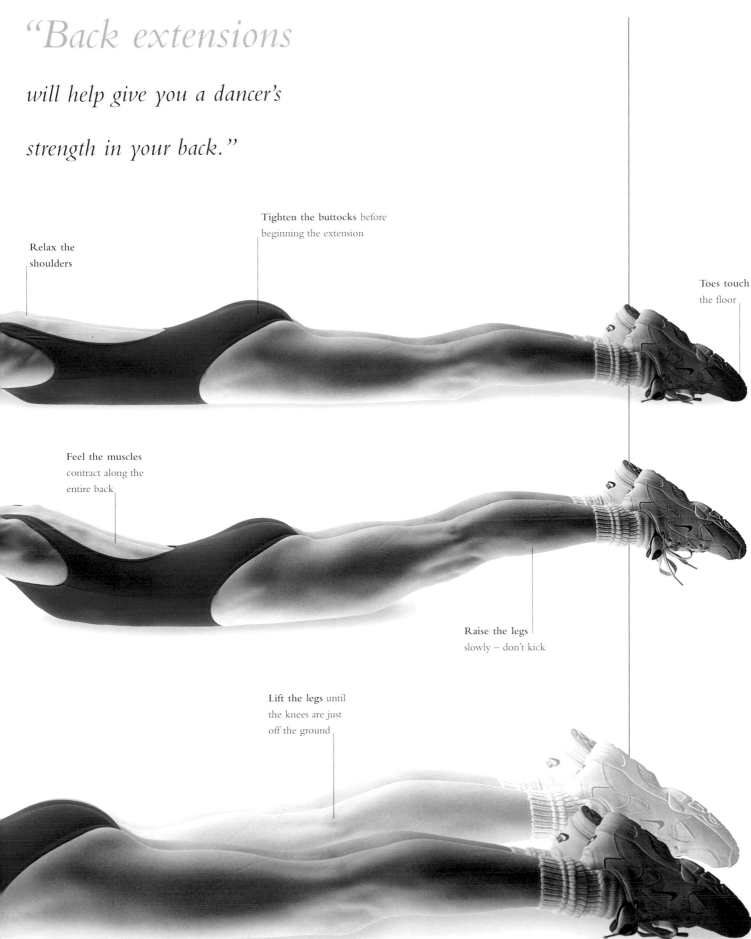

Relax the
shoulders

Tighten the buttocks before
beginning the extension

Toes touch
the floor

Feel the muscles
contract along the
entire back

Raise the legs
slowly – don't kick

Lift the legs until
the knees are just
off the ground

67

Chair Dips

Chair dips offer an excellent alternative to the more usual push-ups because they work a wider combination of muscles. This is a very safe way of exercising the latissimus dorsi in the back, as well as the triceps and pectorals, since it provides some traction for the spine. Chair dips will improve muscle tone in the torso and help firm the back of the upper arms.

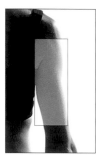

THE TRICEPS MUSCLE, situated along the back of the upper arm, crosses both the shoulder joint and the elbow.

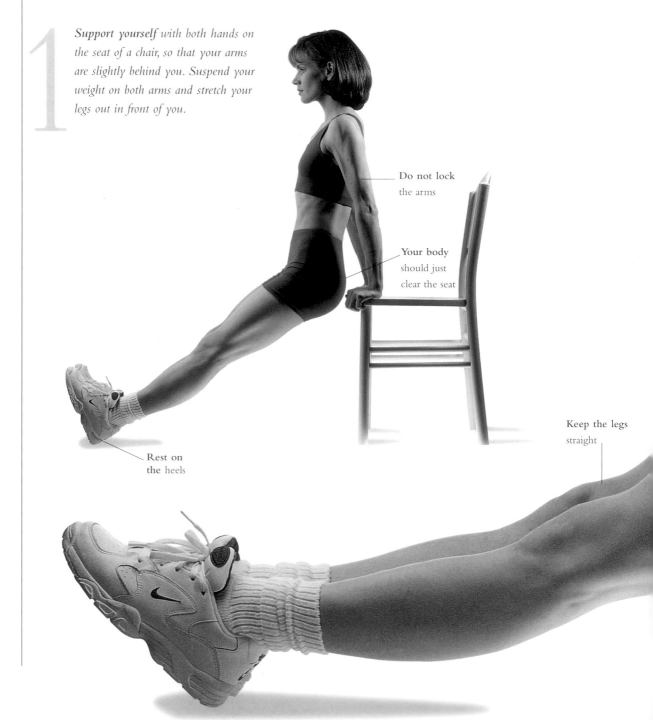

1 **Support yourself** with both hands on the seat of a chair, so that your arms are slightly behind you. Suspend your weight on both arms and stretch your legs out in front of you.

Do not lock the arms

Your body should just clear the seat

Keep the legs straight

Rest on the heels

CAUTION

Do not lower yourself too far at first, or you might strain the shoulder joint.

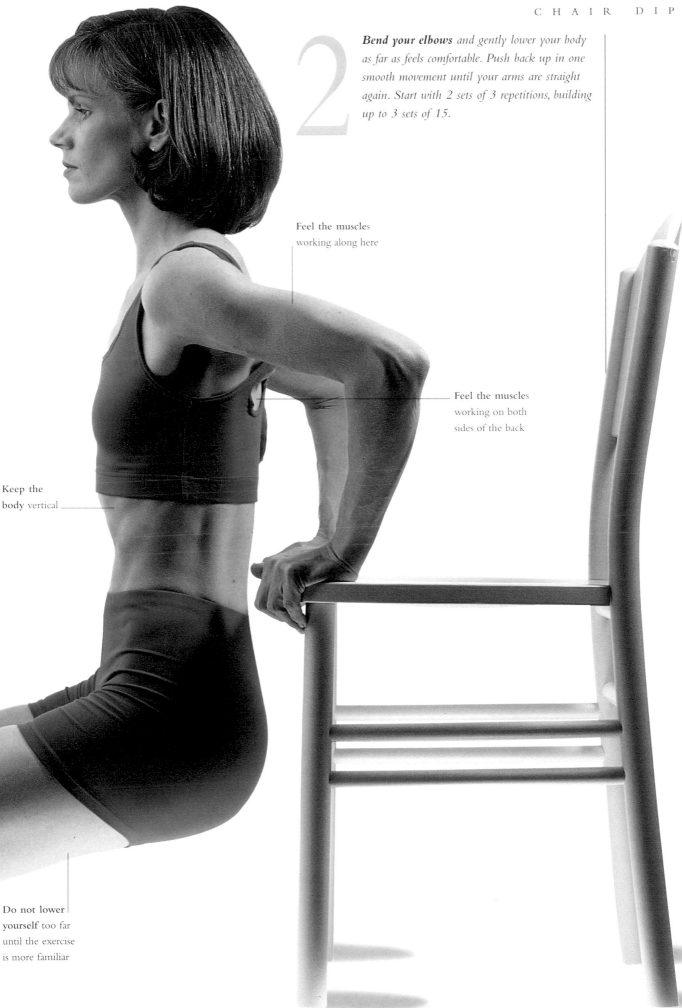

2 **Bend your elbows** and gently lower your body as far as feels comfortable. Push back up in one smooth movement until your arms are straight again. Start with 2 sets of 3 repetitions, building up to 3 sets of 15.

Feel the muscles working along here

Feel the muscles working on both sides of the back

Keep the body vertical

Do not lower yourself too far until the exercise is more familiar

Hamstrings

Strong and flexible hamstrings contribute to good posture and work together with the abdominals to protect the lower back. Since most aerobic exercise, such as running and cycling, strengthens the quadriceps at the front of the thigh, selective training of the hamstrings is important to maintain muscular balance.

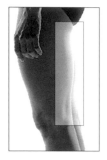

THE HAMSTRINGS is the collective name for the group of muscles in the back of the thigh. They originate at the back of the pelvis and attach below the knee.

Double hamstring

1 *Lie flat on the floor with your arms at your sides for support. Place both heels of your feet on the seat of a chair, with your knees bent at right angles.*

Spread the arms slightly for stability

Knees and hips are bent at a 90° angle

2 *Lift your pelvis high off the floor by pushing your weight down onto your heels. Hold the position briefly.*

Feet rest on the heels

3 *Move your pelvis up and down, without letting your bottom touch the ground. Rest and repeat. Start with 2 sets of 3 repetitions, building up to 3 sets of 7.*

Keep the arms flat on the ground

Do not let the bottom touch the floor

CAUTION

Do not attempt too many repetitions until you are accustomed to this exercise.

One-legged hamstring

You can progress to this exercise once you are able to complete the double hamstring with ease. Lie as before, but with your right heel on the seat of the chair and your left leg pointing upward. Lift your pelvis high off the floor by pushing down through your right heel, and move up and down as before, without letting your body touch the ground. Lower yourself down and repeat with your other leg. Start with 2 sets of 6 repetitions, building up to 3 sets of 14.

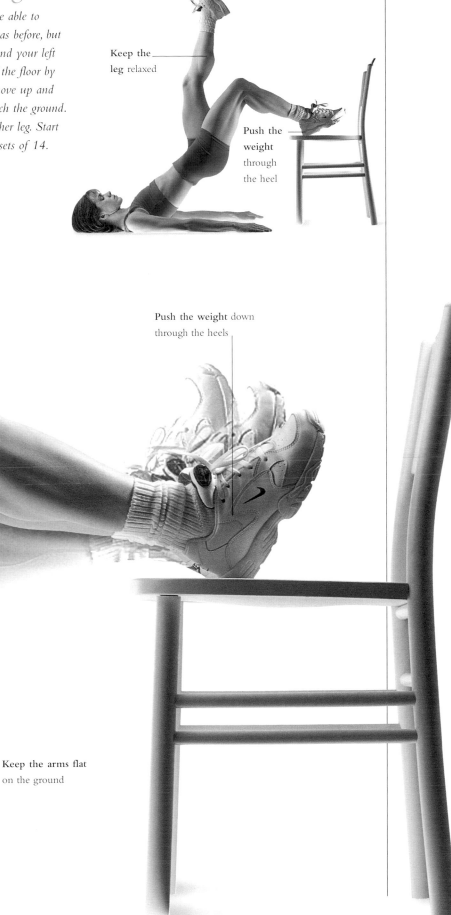

Keep the leg relaxed

Push the weight through the heel

Push the weight down through the heels

Keep the arms flat on the ground

Biceps

This exercise can be performed in one of three ways. The inclined chin-up and the arm-curl (with its elastic resistance) offer easier alternatives to the chin-up for working the biceps and brachialis muscles, and women may find these versions easier to execute. For the chin-ups, you will need a bar or tree branch, and for the arm-curl, an elastic exercise band (see pages 52 – 53).

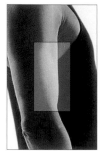

THE BICEPS AND BRACHIALIS are the muscles opposing the triceps. Together, they provide bulk and strength in the upper arm.

Chin-up

Underhand grip

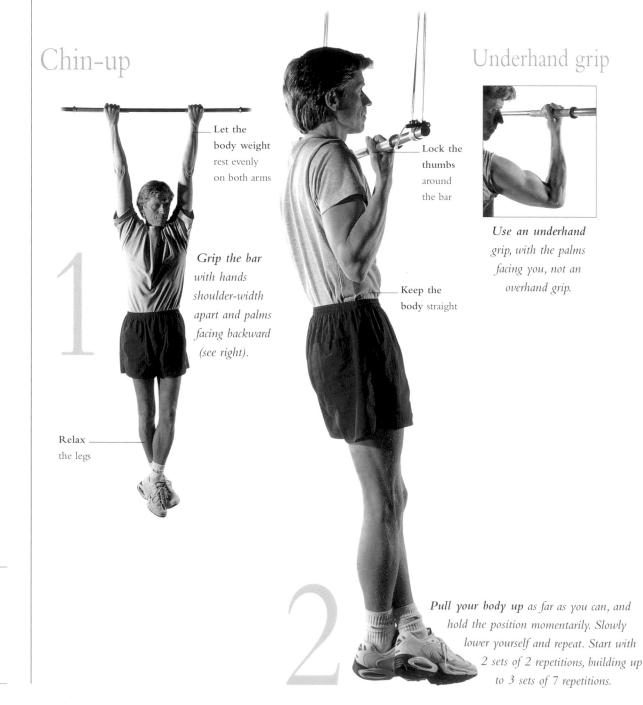

1

Let the body weight rest evenly on both arms

Grip the bar with hands shoulder-width apart and palms facing backward (see right).

Relax the legs

Lock the thumbs around the bar

Keep the body straight

Use an underhand grip, with the palms facing you, not an overhand grip.

2

Pull your body up as far as you can, and hold the position momentarily. Slowly lower yourself and repeat. Start with 2 sets of 2 repetitions, building up to 3 sets of 7 repetitions.

CAUTION

If chin-ups feel too hard, switch to the arm-curls until you have increased your strength.

Inclined chin-up

1 **Mount the bar** *at waist height. Grasp it with an underhand grip (see opposite), hands shoulder-width apart, keeping your body straight and your heels on the ground.*

Keep the body straight

Heels are hip-width apart

Check that the body is in line

2 **Pull yourself up** *as high as possible and hold the position momentarily, before slowly lowering yourself. Start with 2 sets of 2 repetitions, building up to 3 sets of 7 repetitions.*

Arm-curl

1 **Place your right foot** *slightly in front of your left and hook the elastic beneath it. Hold the elastic in your right hand, with your elbow bent and the elastic tight enough to give slight resistance.*

Part the legs for stability

Elastic exercise band

Adjust elastic tension so that the repetitions are just possible

Hold the back straight

Ensure that the elbow is close to the body

2 **Bend your elbow** *and pull the elastic up to your shoulder. Hold the position briefly before slowly lowering your arm. Start with 2 sets of 6 repetitions on each arm, building up to 3 sets of 10 repetitions.*

CAUTION

Do not let the elastic slip from beneath the foot.

73

Arabesque

This position is one of the most common used in ballet. Here, we borrow it from the dance class and adapt it for use in strength training. Ballet technique is not always appropriate for nondancers, but the combination of turn-out and lift in the arabesque is particularly effective in working the gluteal muscles and firming the buttocks.

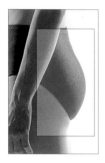

THE GLUTEAL MUSCLES make up the bulk of the buttocks. They connect the pelvis and the femur bone in the thigh.

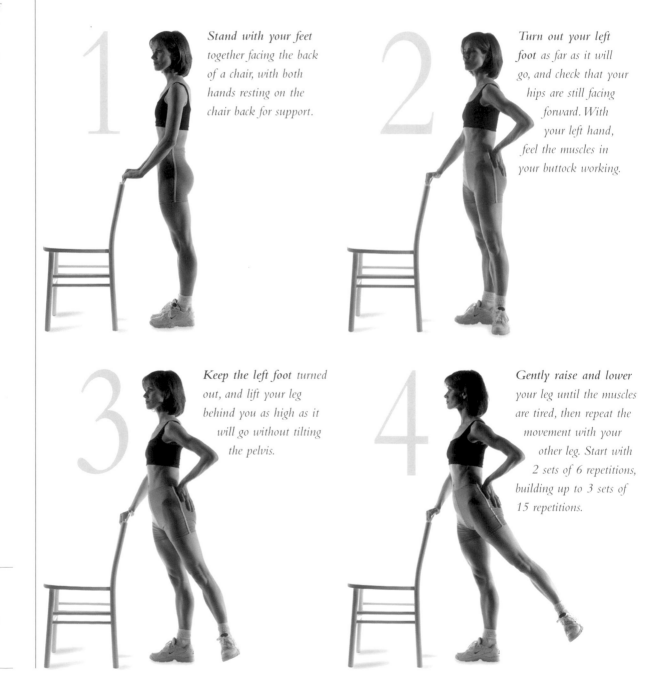

1 *Stand with your feet together facing the back of a chair, with both hands resting on the chair back for support.*

2 *Turn out your left foot as far as it will go, and check that your hips are still facing forward. With your left hand, feel the muscles in your buttock working.*

3 *Keep the left foot turned out, and lift your leg behind you as high as it will go without tilting the pelvis.*

4 *Gently raise and lower your leg until the muscles are tired, then repeat the movement with your other leg. Start with 2 sets of 6 repetitions, building up to 3 sets of 15 repetitions.*

CAUTION

Do not lift the foot too high, or you may strain the lower back.

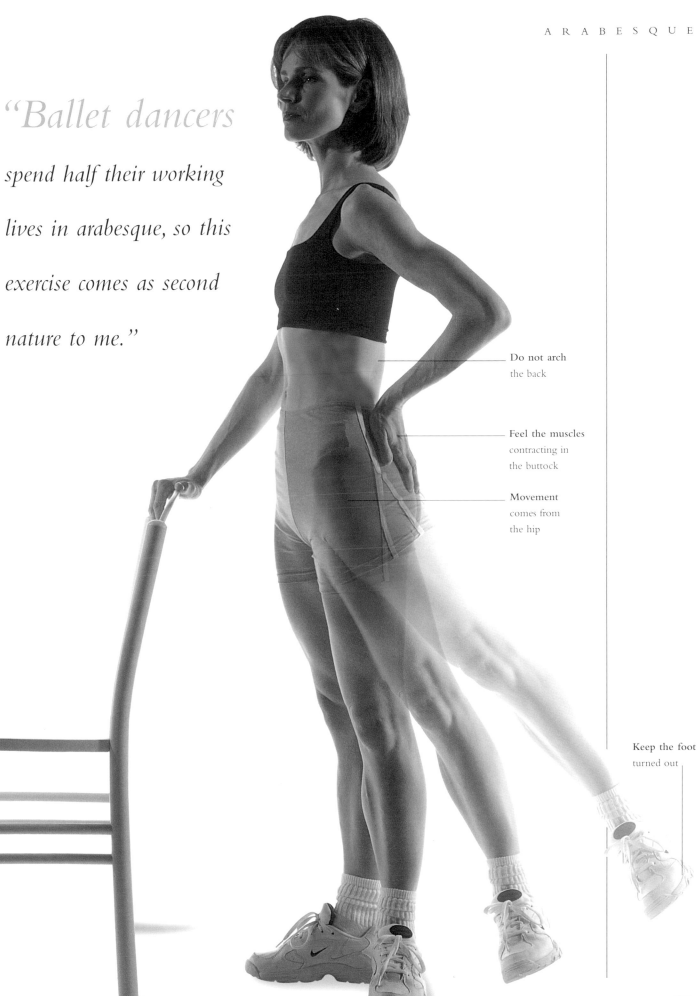

"Ballet dancers spend half their working lives in arabesque, so this exercise comes as second nature to me."

Do not arch
the back

Feel the muscles
contracting in
the buttock

Movement
comes from
the hip

Keep the foot
turned out

Inner Thigh

The adductors are the muscles on the inside of the thighs that bring the legs together – you feel them work when you cross one leg over the other. This exercise has a strong aesthetic factor, since it helps firm the inner thighs. It also develops the specific strength needed in sports such as football, skiing, and rollerblading.

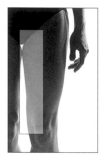

THE ADDUCTORS stretch between the knee and the pelvis, on the inside of the thigh.

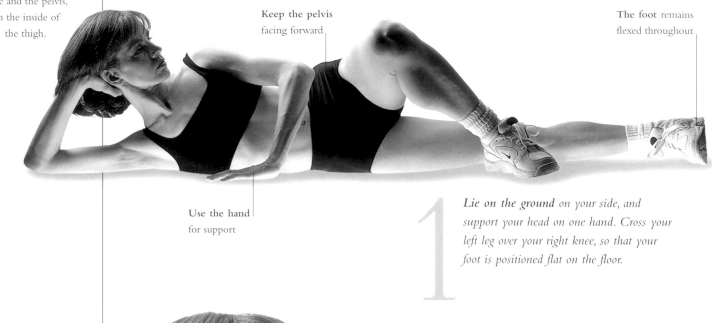

Keep the pelvis facing forward

The foot remains flexed throughout

Use the hand for support

1 *Lie on the ground on your side, and support your head on one hand. Cross your left leg over your right knee, so that your foot is positioned flat on the floor.*

Do not twist the torso

"*Feel the muscles*

working by resting your hand on

your leg from time to time."

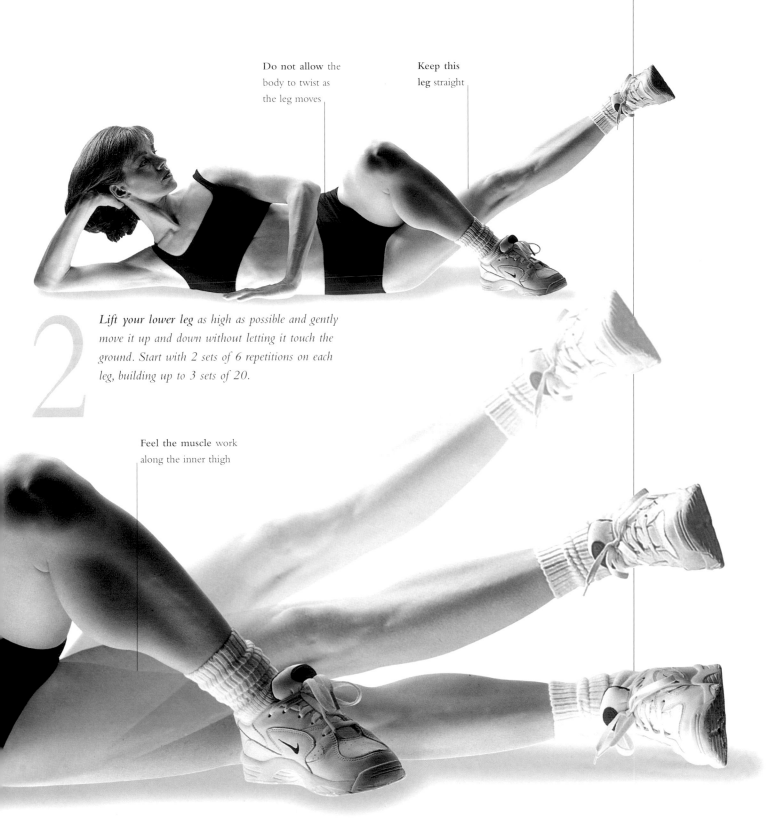

Do not allow the
body to twist as
the leg moves

Keep this
leg straight

2

Lift your lower leg *as high as possible and gently
move it up and down without letting it touch the
ground. Start with 2 sets of 6 repetitions on each
leg, building up to 3 sets of 20.*

Feel the muscle work
along the inner thigh

Deltoid

A large, triangular muscle, the deltoid covers the shoulder and is used to lift the arms. By lifting the arm sideways against elastic resistance, you work as much of the muscle as possible in one movement. This exercise tones the shoulders, strengthens the arms, and improves the look of the upper body. You will need an elastic exercise band (see pages 52 – 53).

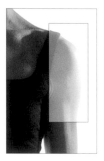

THE DELTOID MUSCLE originates from the collar bone and shoulder blade and attaches to the humerus, the bone of the upper arm.

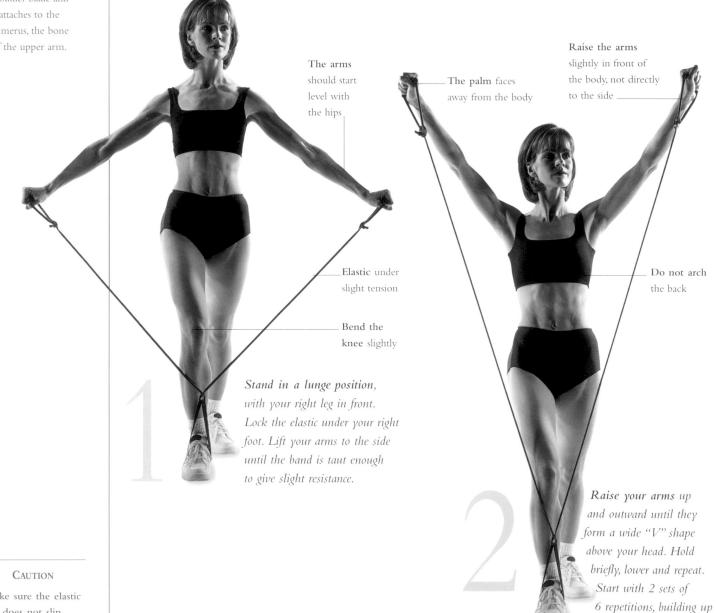

The arms should start level with the hips

Elastic under slight tension

Bend the knee slightly

Stand in a lunge position, with your right leg in front. Lock the elastic under your right foot. Lift your arms to the side until the band is taut enough to give slight resistance.

The palm faces away from the body

Raise the arms slightly in front of the body, not directly to the side

Do not arch the back

Raise your arms up and outward until they form a wide "V" shape above your head. Hold briefly, lower and repeat. Start with 2 sets of 6 repetitions, building up to 3 sets of 10 repetitions.

CAUTION
Make sure the elastic does not slip.

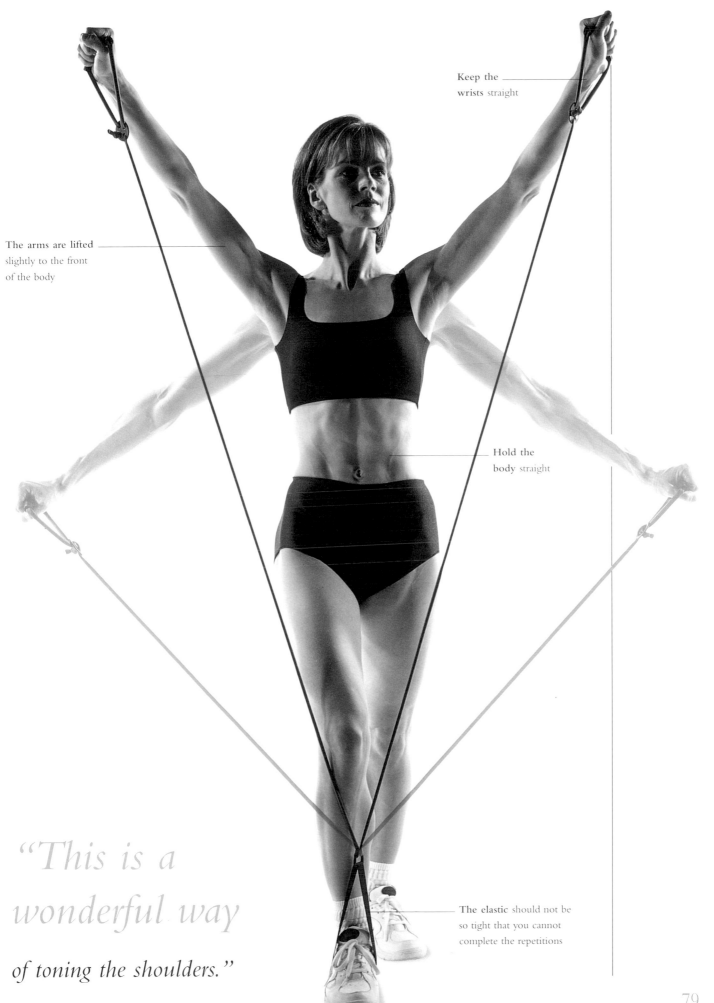

Keep the
wrists straight

The **arms are lifted**
slightly to the front
of the body

Hold the
body straight

The **elastic** should not be
so tight that you cannot
complete the repetitions

"This is a
wonderful way

of toning the shoulders."

Stretches

STRETCHES

THE STRETCHES

Stretch both sides of
your body equally

■

INNER THIGH
STRETCH

■

HIP FLEXOR
STRETCH

■

HAMSTRING
STRETCH

■

UPPER AND LOWER
CALF STRETCH

■

SIDE STRETCH

■

CAT/HANGING
(WHOLE-BODY)
STRETCH

Never underestimate the value of stretching: it increases muscle length and flexibility, and long, supple muscles are less prone to injury. Short muscles, however strong they are, will always be a source of problems because they cannot cope with such a wide range of movement. Stretching after your workout is especially effective, because aerobic exercise raises your body temperature, and the connective tissue of muscles is much more elastic when it is warm.

When practiced correctly, stretching should be a pleasant, not a painful experience. Take the stretch position gently, breathe in, and then sink deeper into it as you breathe out. Focus on the muscle you are stretching and feel it relax as you hold the position for a count of 10. Do the exercises in the order in which they are listed, and be sure to stretch both sides of the body equally. You should repeat the stretches as instructed.

Do not bounce: it stimulates a protective mechanism in the muscle that causes it to tighten as a defense against injury. Your flexibility will increase over a matter of weeks, not overnight, so never try to force your body; stretching is one of those things you just can't rush.

Inner Thigh

The adductors are a group of muscles on the inside of the thigh that are used to bring the legs together. A healthy back depends on a good range of movement in the hip joint, and if the adductors are tight, they can limit mobility.

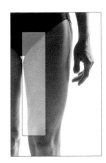

THE ADDUCTORS stretch between the knee and the pelvis and are located on the inside of the thigh.

1

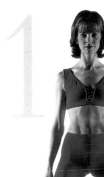

Stand with your legs wide apart, feet facing forward, and your arms hanging at your sides.

Legs
wide apart

Do not drop
the head

Body weight
rests on the
hands

Feel the
stretch along
the inner thigh

Bend the knee

2

Bend your left knee and bring your body weight over it, so that your hands rest on the thigh. Hold this position for a count of 10, before returning to the starting position and repeating with your right leg.

CAUTION

Do not lean forward. Push against the thigh to ensure that you do not round the back.

81

Hip Flexor

The psoas muscle, commonly called the hip flexor, lifts the leg in front of the body – an action used, for instance, in running and walking. Due to its complex relationship with the hip and spine, it rarely gets to stretch out fully. A tight psoas pulls on the lower spine, contributing to back pain. Combining flexible psoas with strong abdominal muscles protects the lower back.

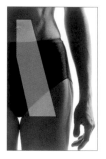

THE PSOAS MUSCLE
(the "p" is silent)
runs between the
femur, or thigh bone,
and the lower spine.

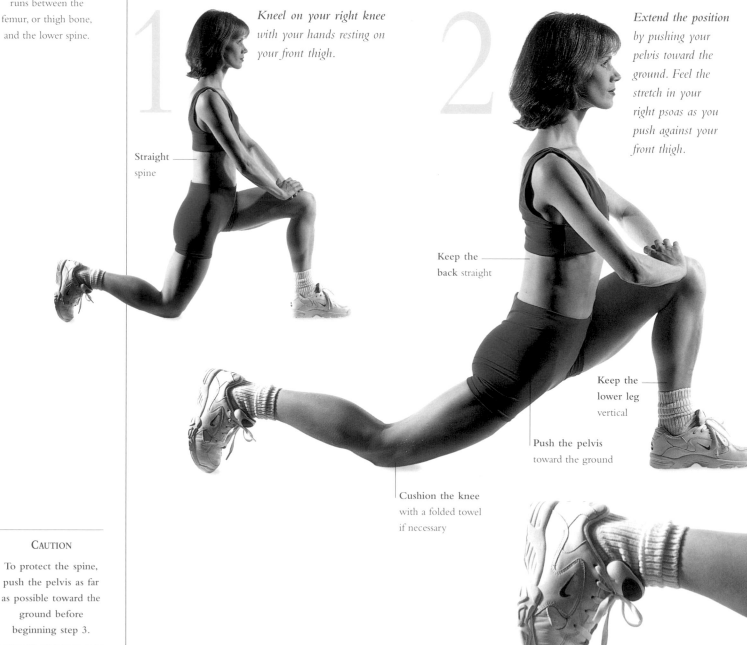

1 *Kneel on your right knee with your hands resting on your front thigh.*

Straight spine

2 *Extend the position by pushing your pelvis toward the ground. Feel the stretch in your right psoas as you push against your front thigh.*

Keep the back straight

Keep the lower leg vertical

Push the pelvis toward the ground

Cushion the knee with a folded towel if necessary

CAUTION

To protect the spine, push the pelvis as far as possible toward the ground before beginning step 3.

82

Stretch the arm
to form an arc

3

Balance yourself *with your left
hand, and raise your right arm up
and backward to complete the stretch.
Hold for a count of 10, then return
to the starting position and
repeat on the other side.*

Arch the spine
gently backward

"*Fine-tune* all of these

stretches to maximize their

effectiveness for your

own physique."

Feel the stretch
along here

Front Thigh

The rectus femoris is one of the four quadriceps muscles in the front of the thigh. Of the four, it is the only one that crosses the hip and knee joints. Any action that involves lifting a straight leg in front of you – kicking a ball, for instance – will activate the rectus femoris. If it is tight, it may tilt the pelvis forward, causing problems in the lower back.

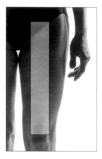

THE RECTUS FEMORIS MUSCLE is located along the front thigh and stretches from the knee to the hip.

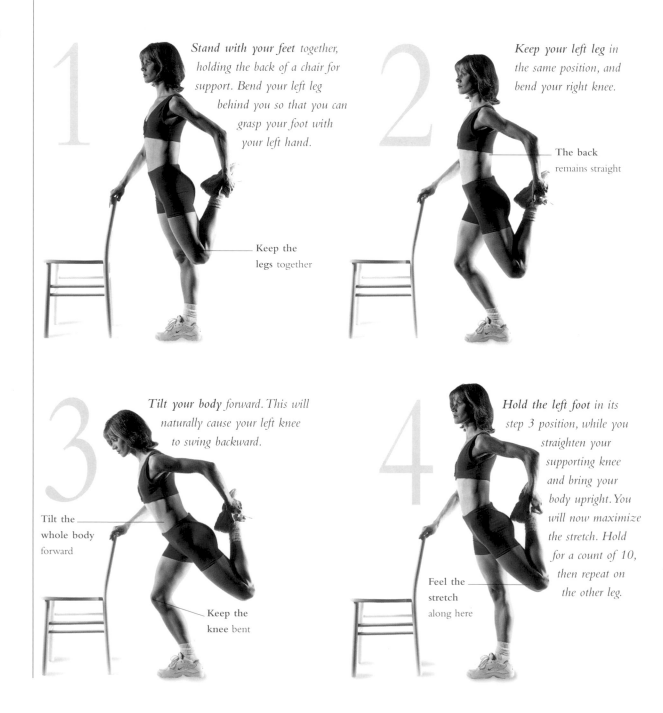

1 *Stand with your feet* together, holding the back of a chair for support. Bend your left leg behind you so that you can grasp your foot with your left hand.

Keep the legs together

2 *Keep your left leg in* the same position, and bend your right knee.

The back remains straight

3 *Tilt your body* forward. This will naturally cause your left knee to swing backward.

Tilt the whole body forward

Keep the knee bent

4 *Hold the left foot in its* step 3 position, while you straighten your supporting knee and bring your body upright. You will now maximize the stretch. Hold for a count of 10, then repeat on the other leg.

Feel the stretch along here

Hamstrings

The group of muscles in the back of the thigh is collectively known as the hamstrings. They are used to bend the knee and lift the leg behind the body. Tight hamstrings are easily injured and can also be an indirect cause of back pain.

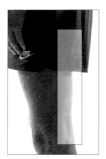

THE HAMSTRINGS originate at the back of the pelvis and attach below the knee.

Do not drop the head

Do not round the upper back

Bend the knee slightly

Bend from the hip

Rest the foot on the heel, not the Achilles' tendon

Feel the stretch along here

Lift your left leg, and place your foot on the back of a chair at approximately waist height. Bend forward from the hip, keeping your eyes focused ahead of you. Hold the stretch for a count of 10, then relax and repeat with your right leg.

CAUTION

To avoid stressing the sciatic nerve, keep the raised foot relaxed the knee slightly bent, and look straight ahead.

Upper Calf

The calf has two major muscles: the gastrocnemius and the soleus. The gastrocnemius is the rounded, upper part that provides the powerful push-off used in walking, running, and jumping. If tight, it can lead to problems with the Achilles' tendon to which it is connected and may distort the alignment of the foot.

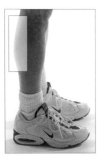

THE GASTROCNEMIUS MUSCLE is in the upper part of the calf. It originates at the femur and inserts at the heel.

1 *Stand close to a solid wall, with the ball of your right foot against it, so that only your heel touches the ground.*

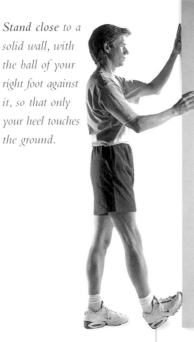

Move toward the wall

Lock the heel into the ground

2 *Keeping your front knee straight, push forward, so your hips move toward the wall and the heel of your hind foot lifts slightly off the floor. Hold for a count of 10, then repeat on your left leg.*

Ensure the knee is straight

CAUTION

Move gently from step 1 to step 2, since this technique can generate considerable force.

Lower Calf

The soleus is a broad, flat muscle in the lower part of the calf. Unlike the other stretches shown, which involve muscles crossing two joints, the soleus is a one-joint muscle, crossing only the ankle. One-joint muscles do not usually cause problems, but the soleus needs special attention since it works so closely with the gastrocnemius.

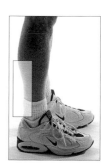

THE SOLEUS MUSCLE originates in the bones of the lower leg and combines with the gastrocnemius to form the Achilles' tendon.

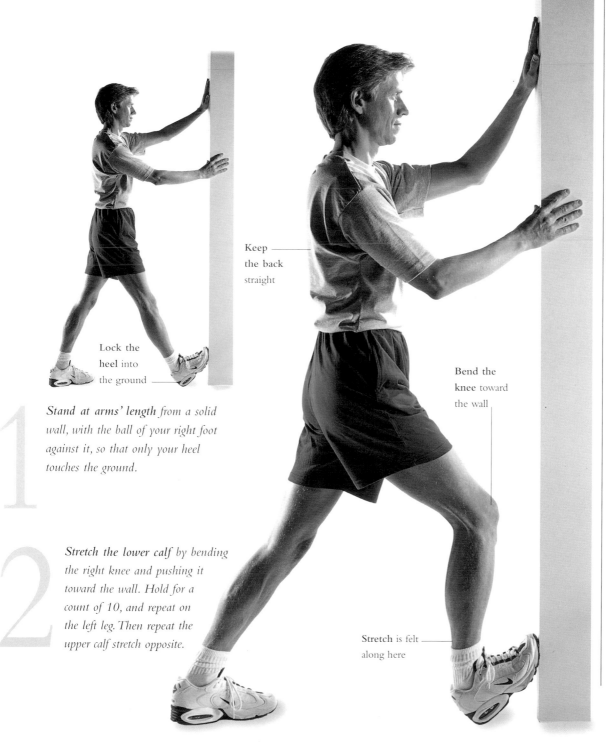

Keep the back straight

Lock the heel into the ground

Bend the knee toward the wall

Stretch is felt along here

1 *Stand at arms' length from a solid wall, with the ball of your right foot against it, so that only your heel touches the ground.*

2 *Stretch the lower calf by bending the right knee and pushing it toward the wall. Hold for a count of 10, and repeat on the left leg. Then repeat the upper calf stretch opposite.*

87

Side Stretch

This stretch elongates the entire side of the body, from the knee through to the fingertips. Its primary function is to stretch the muscles on the outside of the hip, but this is an all-purpose exercise that also targets the muscles that bend the body to the side and the muscles that lie between the ribs.

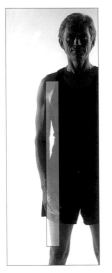

THE TENSOR FASCIAE LATAE and the OBLIQUE ABDOMINAL MUSCLES lie at the side of the body. THE INTERCOSTAL MUSCLES lie between the ribs.

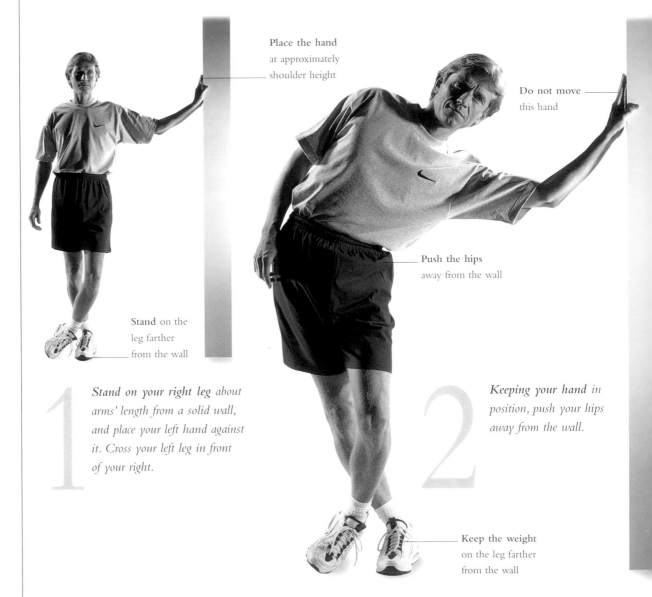

Place the hand at approximately shoulder height

Stand on the leg farther from the wall

1 *Stand on your right leg about arms' length from a solid wall, and place your left hand against it. Cross your left leg in front of your right.*

Do not move this hand

Push the hips away from the wall

Keep the weight on the leg farther from the wall

2 *Keeping your hand in position, push your hips away from the wall.*

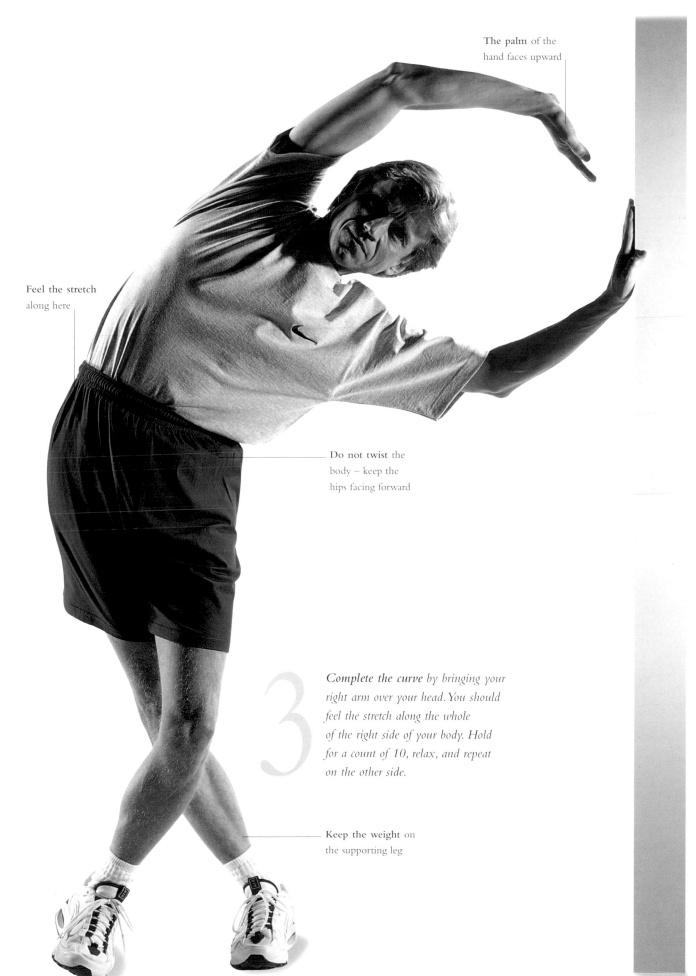

The palm of the hand faces upward

Feel the stretch along here

Do not twist the body – keep the hips facing forward

3

Complete the curve by bringing your right arm over your head. You should feel the stretch along the whole of the right side of your body. Hold for a count of 10, relax, and repeat on the other side.

Keep the weight on the supporting leg

Cat Stretch

The spine is made up of 24 individual vertebrae held together by muscles, ligaments, and disks. A healthy spine relies on normal mobility between each of these bones. Where this is limited, back problems can arise. The cat stretch is an excellent way to mobilize your spine safely and so guard against back problems.

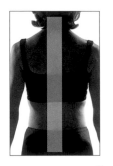

THE VERTEBRAE run all the way down the the back, from the skull to the tail bone.

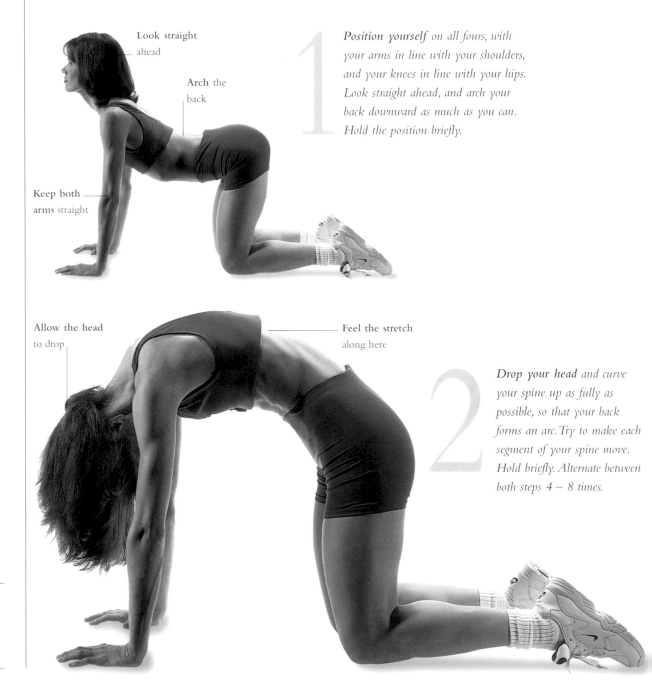

Look straight ahead

Arch the back

Keep both arms straight

1

Position yourself on all fours, with your arms in line with your shoulders, and your knees in line with your hips. Look straight ahead, and arch your back downward as much as you can. Hold the position briefly.

Allow the head to drop

Feel the stretch along here

2

Drop your head and curve your spine up as fully as possible, so that your back forms an arc. Try to make each segment of your spine move. Hold briefly. Alternate between both steps 4 – 8 times.

CAUTION

To avoid neck injury, keep the head straight in step 1.

Hanging Stretch

Ever since humans began to walk upright, the spine has been subject to the negative effects of gravity. The hanging stretch helps to counteract these by providing traction for the spine as well as the shoulder joints. If you do not have a suitable bar (see pages 52 – 53), use a sturdy branch on a tree instead.

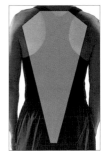

THE SPINAL COLUMN is made up of the vertebrae and encloses the spinal cord, which it protects.

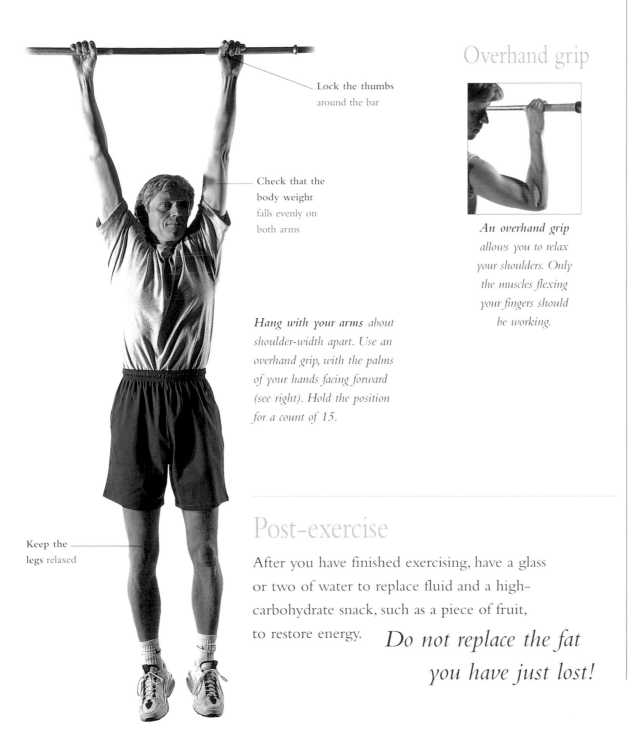

Lock the thumbs around the bar

Check that the body weight falls evenly on both arms

Hang with your arms about shoulder-width apart. Use an overhand grip, with the palms of your hands facing forward (see right). Hold the position for a count of 15.

Keep the legs relaxed

Overhand grip

An overhand grip allows you to relax your shoulders. Only the muscles flexing your fingers should be working.

Post-exercise

After you have finished exercising, have a glass or two of water to replace fluid and a high-carbohydrate snack, such as a piece of fruit, to restore energy. *Do not replace the fat you have just lost!*

Glossary

Aerobic Exercise: Low-intensity, high-duration exercise during which energy is supplied using oxygen. Aerobic endurance exercise is the only type of exercise that causes fat to be broken down and used directly as the main source of energy.

Amino Acids: Organic compounds necessary in the formation of proteins. Essential amino acids cannot be manufactured by the body and must be obtained from food.

Anaerobic Exercise: High-intensity, short-duration exercise that is fueled by carbohydrates and doesn't utilize oxygen.

Blood-sugar Level: The concentration of glucose in the blood.

Body Fat: Storage fat that accumulates under the skin.

Calorie: The unit used to indicate the energy value of foods. This energy is used to fuel the body. It is also now measured in joules (1 calorie = 4.19 joules). A "calorie deficit" is when the body uses more calories than the diet provides.

Carbohydrates: The large group of sugars, starches, and dietary fiber that all contain carbon, hydrogen, and oxygen. Carbohydrates are the main source of energy for all body functions and are needed to process other nutrients. They are formed by all green plants, which use the sun to combine carbon dioxide and water into simple sugar molecules. They can also be made in the body.

Cholesterol: A substance found in liver, egg yolk, and some shellfish. It is also made in the human body, mainly in the liver and kidneys. Cholesterol helps to absorb fatty acids and to make vitamin D and various hormones, including the sex hormones, but surplus amounts of it can be dangerous.

Cramp: Prolonged painful contraction of the muscles, often caused by the imbalance of salts in the body, but more often as a result of fatigue, poor posture, or stress.

Diuretic: A substance that increases the flow of urine.

Endorphins: Hormones produced in the brain that have natural pain-relieving qualities. During exercise their production increases, leading to a general sense of well-being.

Energy: Needed for the body to function and be active. All of the body's energy is derived from carbohydrates, protein, and fat.

Enzymes: Proteins that accelerate biological reactions.

Fats: Substances made up of fatty acids that are found in both animals and plants. They provide a concentrated form of energy and can also be stored as body fat.

Glucose: A simple sugar found in certain foods, especially fruits, and is a major source of energy in human and animal metabolism. Glucose can be stored in the liver and muscles as glycogen then converted to glucose and released as needed.

Glycogen: The major carbohydrate stored in animal cells. It is made from glucose and stored chiefly in the liver.

Heart Rate: A measure of cardiac activity, usually expressed as the number of beats per minute.

Hormones: Chemical substances that are released into the bloodstream and act on specific receptor sites in certain parts of the body.

Insulin: Hormone produced by the pancreas that regulates the body's absorption of carbohydrates.

Lactic Acid: A vital substance in the production of energy that is recycled when there is sufficient oxygen available. In anaerobic energy production, it builds up in the cells and limits endurance.

Ligaments: Tough bands of tissue that connect two bones or hold organs in place.

Metabolism: Collective term for chemical changes in living cells by which energy is provided for vital processes like growth and functioning. The "resting metabolic rate" reflects the energy required to keep the body functioning at rest.

Minerals: A group of inorganic substances that occur naturally in the Earth's crust and must be included in the diet. They are important in regulating many bodily functions.

Muscles: Tissues with the ability to contract, causing and allowing movement of the joints.

Obesity: A condition characterized by excessive body fat.

Osteoporosis: A condition in which the density of the bones declines, making them brittle and prone to fracture.

Proteins: Compounds of carbon, hydrogen, oxygen, and nitrogen that provide the raw materials (amino acids) for growth and repair. Proteins form the structural material of muscles, tissues, and organs. In certain circumstances, proteins can be converted into glucose and used for energy.

Repetition: A single, completed movement of an exercise.

Resting Metabolic Rate: See metabolism.

Set: A group of repetitions.

Target Zone: The heart rate range for a specific exercise intensity.

Tendons: Tough bands of connective tissue that unite muscle with another body part, usually bone, and transmit the force that the muscle exerts.

Vertebrae: Bony segments that make up the spinal column.

Vitamins: Organic substances that neither supply energy nor contribute to body mass, yet serve crucial functions in almost all body processes. They must be obtained from the diet.

Index

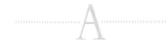

A

abdominal muscles 65, 66, 70, 88
abdominals (strength training) 65
Achilles' tendon 86, 87
adductor muscles 76, 81
aerobic endurance exercise 21, 60–2
　target zones 23, 60
aerobic energy system 21
aerobic exercise 19, 21, 60–2, 92
　adapting for warmup 57
　target zones 23, 60
alcohol 26, 41
amino acids 30–1, 39, 92
anaerobic energy system 20
anaerobic exercise 19, 20, 57, 92
　target zones 23
animal proteins 30
appetite 15, 29
arabesque 74–5
arm-curls 73
arm muscles 68, 72, 78

B

back extensions 66–7
back muscles 66, 68
bagels 33, 43, 49
baked potatoes 44–5
biceps muscles 72
biceps (strength training) 72–3
bike stands 53, 61
bikes & cycling 52–3
　see also cycling
binging 15
biological value 30
blood-sugar levels 14, 29, 54, 92
body fat 92
body fat/muscle comparisons 12, 13, 14, 16
　energy store & source 16, 18, 21, 26
　fat-burning myths 8, 12, 13
　reduction see permanent weight loss
　　& weight control
body wraps 37
brachialis muscles 72
bread 28, 29, 39, 43, 44, 49
breakfast 43

C

caffeine 36, 37, 41
calcium 35
calf muscles 86, 87
calorie content
　body's energy stores 16, 31
　carbohydrates 14, 26, 28
　fats 13, 14, 26
　food-labeling information 26, 40
　protein 26, 30
calorie deficit 14, 26, 92
calorie expenditure 26
　during exercise 14
calories, general information 26–7
carbohydrates 28–9, 92
　body's energy stores 16, 31
　calorie content 14, 26, 28
　effect on blood-sugar levels 14, 29, 54
　food-labeling information 40
　fuel for the brain 12, 16, 28, 30, 31, 54
　fuel for energy systems 9, 20–1, 28
　high-carbohydrate breakfasts 43
　high-carbohydrate diet see high-
　　carbohydrate/low-fat diet
　high-carbohydrate snacks 49, 91
　recommended intake 28, 38–9
cat stretch 90
cereals & grains 28, 31, 34, 39, 43, 45
chair dips 68–9
chin-up bars 53, 56, 72, 73, 91
chin-ups 72–3
cholesterol 32, 33, 92
clothing
　exercise 52
　plastic sweat wear 13, 37
cold-weather clothing 52
complete proteins 30
complex carbohydrates 28, 29, 40
cookies 33, 49
cooking techniques, recommended
　34, 38, 46, 47
cool-down 63
cool-weather clothing 52
cramp 92
cross-country skiing 61
cycling & bikes 52, 53, 57, 61, 62
　as aerobic exercise 61, 62
　as warmup 57
　and wind chill 53

D

dairy products, nutritional content
　30, 32, 33, 34, 35, 39
dehydration 36, 37
deltoid (strength training)
　78–9
deltoid muscles 78
desserts 47
dietary fiber 29, 40
dieting see weight loss
diets & dieting
　high-protein/low-carbohydrate
　31, 39
　myths 7, 8, 10, 12–3
　recommended see high-carbohydrate/
　　low-fat diet
　yo-yo 7, 8
digestion 13, 27, 54
dinner 46–7
diuretics 92
double hamstring
　(strength training) 70
drinks 36, 37, 41, 54
duration, exercise 19

E

eating pattern, recommended 41
elastic exercise bands 53, 56, 73
endorphins 15, 92
endurance exercise see aerobic
　endurance exercise
energy 92
　measurement see calories
　storage & use 13, 16, 20–1, 27, 54
　　protein conversion into glucose 12,
　　27, 30, 31
energy drinks 54
English muffins 49
enzymes 13, 92
equipment, exercise 52–3, 56
erector spinae muscles 66
essential amino acids 30, 39, 92
essential fatty acids 32
exercise
　calorie expenditure 14

exercise *continued*
  effect on appetite 15
  effect on metabolic rate 14, 27
  effect on muscles 12, 15, 16
  equipment, clothing & footwear
    52–3, 56
  increasing general activity levels, 55, 62
  intensity & duration 19, 22
  myths 12, 13
  osteoporosis prevention 15, 35
  post-exercise advice 91
  pre-exercise plan 55
  role in weight loss & control 14, 15, 18
  when & when not to exercise 54
  see also individual types of exercise
    by name, such as aerobic exercise,
    strength training

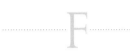

fat-burning myths 8, 12, 13
fat content
  calculating 40
  carbohydrate foods 29
  food-labeling information 40
  protein foods 30, 31
fat-soluble vitamins 32, 34
fats 32–3, 92
  in the body *see* body fat
  calorie content 13, 14, 26
  cause of obesity 16, 39
  low-fat diet see high carbohydrate/
    low-fat diet
  recommended intake 32, 39
fatty acids 32, 92
feces, water loss in 37
fiber, dietary 29, 40
first aid 58
fish 30, 32, 35, 39, 46
flat feet 53
flour 28, 29
fluid balance 36
food
  as energy source 16, 26
  food groups *see individually by name,*
    such as carbohydrates
  food-labeling information 26, 40
  water content 36
food combining 13
foot types 53
footwear 52, 53, 56
front thigh, stretch exercise 84
fructose 28
fruit & vegetables
  in meals and snacks 43–8, 91

nutritional content 28, 29, 30, 34, 35
recommended intake 34, 38
water content 36

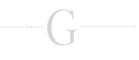

gastrocnemius muscles 86
glucose 28, 92
  protein conversion into 12, 27, 30, 31
gluteal muscles 74
glycogen 28, 92
grains & cereals 28, 31, 34, 39, 43, 45
great protein myth 31
grips, on chin-up bars 72, 91

H

hamstrings 57, 70, 85
  strength training 70–1
  stretch exercise 85
hanging stretch 91
heart activity during exercise 20, 21, 57
heart rate 22–3, 60, 92
helmets, cycle 52
high-arched feet 53
high-carbohydrate/low-fat diet
  dietary guidelines 38–9
  meal guidelines & suggestions 42–9
  replacements for high-fat foods 33
  role in weight loss & control 9, 14,
    15, 18, 24
  seven-point plan 41
  see also individual food groups by
    name, such as carbohydrates
high-intensity exercise *see* anaerobic
  exercise
high-protein/low-carbohydrate diet 31, 39
hip flexor (stretch exercise) 82–3
hip flexor muscles 82
hormones 92
hybrid bikes 52
hydrogenated fats 33

IJK

ICE (ice, compression, elevation) 58
inclined chin-up 73
ingredients lists 40
injuries & injury prevention 55, 57, 58, 59

inner thighs
  strength training 76–7
  stretch exercise 81
insensible perspiration 37
insulin 54, 92
intensity, exercise 19, 22
intercostal muscles 88
interval training 60
iron 35
jogging & running 55, 57, 60, 62, 63
kcals or kcalories 26, 40
kjoules or kilojoules 26, 40

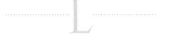

labels, food-labeling information 26, 40
lactic acid 20, 57, 92
lactose 28
latissimus dorsi muscles 68
LDL cholesterol 32
lean tissue 92
ligaments 92
light stretch 58–9
long-duration exercise *see* aerobic
  endurance exercise; aerobic exercise
low-fat diet *see* high-carbohydrate/
  low-fat diet
low-intensity exercise *see* aerobic endurance
  exercise; aerobic exercise
lower calf (stretch exercise) 87
lunch 44–5
lung capacity 21

M

marinades 47
maximum heart rate 23
meals
  guidelines & suggestions 42–9
  recommended eating pattern 41
  timing before exercise 54
meat
  nutritional content 30, 31, 32, 33,
    34, 35, 39
  recommended cooking methods 46–7
metabolism & metabolic rate 13, 14, 27, 92
minerals 26, 29, 34, 35, 92
mini trampolines 62
"miracle diets," myths 7, 8, 10, 13
moderate-intensity exercise *see* aerobic
  exercise
monitors, heart-rate 23, 53

monounsaturated fats 22

mountain bikes 52

muscles 16, 92
　　body fat/muscle comparisons 12, 13,
　　　　14, 16
　　cool-down 63
　　effect of exercise 12, 15, 16
　　effect of stretching 58–9
　　energy use 13, 16
　　loss 12, 13, 27, 31
　　strength training 64–79
　　stretches 58–9, 80–91
　　warming up 57, 59
　　see also individual muscle groups by name,
　　　　such as abdominal muscles

myths
　　dieting & weight loss 7, 8, 10,
　　　　12–3
　　great protein myth 31, 92

N O

neutral feet 53

nutritional tables 26, 40

obesity & overweight 7, 16, 39, 92

oils 32, 33

omega-3 fatty acids 32

one-legged hamstring (strength training) 71

osteoporosis 15, 35, 92

overhand grip, hanging stretch 91

oxygen use during exercise 20–1, 57

P

pasta 28, 29, 31, 39, 45, 46

pectoral muscles 68

permanent weight loss & weight control
　　diet/exercise combination 9, 14, 16, 18
　　health & other benefits 15
　　practical methods 14
　　recommended diet see high-carbohydrate/
　　　　low-fat diet

perspiration
　　insensible 37
　　see also sweating

pita bread 49

pizza 47

plant protein 30–1

plastic sweat wear 13, 37

polyunsaturated fats 22–3

popcorn 49

post-exercise advice 91

potatoes 28, 31, 39, 44–5, 47

poultry 30, 31, 39, 47

pre-exercise plan 55

pretzels 49

pronating feet 53

protein 30–1, 92
　　breakdown products 37
　　calorie content 26, 30
　　conversion into glucose 12, 27, 30, 31
　　food-labeling information 40
　　great protein myth 31, 92
　　high-protein/low-carbohydrate diet
　　　　31, 39
　　in muscles 16
　　recommended intake 30, 39

psoas muscles 82

pulse rate 22–3

Q R

quadriceps muscles 70, 84

rectus femoris muscles 84

refined sugars 29, 40, 54

repetitions 64, 92

resting metabolic rate 27, 92

rice 28, 29, 31, 39, 45, 46

rice cakes 49

rowing 62

running & jogging 55, 57, 60, 62, 63

S

salads 45

salt 35, 40

sandwiches 44, 49

saturated fats 32–3, 40

scones 49

sets 92

shock absorbency, shoes 53

shoes 52, 53, 56

short-duration exercise see anaerobic
　　exercise

side stretch 88–9

simple carbohydrates (simple sugars) 28

skiing, cross-country 61

snacks 33, 48–9, 91

socks 52

sodium 35, 40

soleus muscles 87

soups 45

soybeans 31

spine & spinal column 66, 90, 91

spot-reducing 12, 13

starches 28, 29, 40

starting levels, pre-exercise plan 55

strength training 64
　　abdominals 65
　　arabesque 74–5
　　arm-curls 73
　　back extensions 66–7
　　biceps 72–3
　　chair dips 68–9
　　chin-ups 72–3
　　deltoid 78–9
　　hamstrings 70–1
　　inclined chin-up 73
　　inner thigh 76–7

stretches 58–9, 80
　　cat stretch 90
　　front thigh 84
　　hamstrings 85
　　hanging stretch 91
　　hip flexor 82–3
　　inner thigh 81
　　light stretch 58–9
　　lower calf 87
　　side stretch 88–9
　　upper calf 86

sucrose 28

sugar content
　　drinks 36, 54
　　food-labeling information 40
　　reduced-fat foods 33

sugars 28–9, 40

supinating feet 53

sweating 37
　　"breathable" clothing 52
　　salt loss 35
　　sweat pants 13, 37

swimming 62

T

target zones (target heart rate) 23,
　　60, 92

tendons 92

tensor fasciae latae muscles 88

thigh muscles 57, 76, 81, 84
　　strength training 76–7
　　stretch exercises 81, 84
　　see also hamstrings

tofu 30, 35, 39

trampolining 62

triceps muscles 68, 72

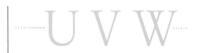

U V W

underhand grip, chin-ups 72
unrefined carbohydrates 28–9
unsaturated fats 32–3, 39, 40
upper calf (stretch exercise) 86
urea 37
urine, water loss in 37
vegetables & fruit
  in meals and snacks 43–8, 91
  nutritional content 28, 29, 30, 34, 35
  recommended intake 34, 38

water content 36
vertebrae 66, 90, 91, 92
vitamins 26, 29, 32, 34–5, 92
walking 55, 57, 60, 61
warmup 57
warm-weather clothing 52
water 36–7
  in muscles 16
  recommended intake 13, 36, 41, 91
  zero calorie content 13, 26
water loss
  during dieting & weight loss 13, 18, 37
  normal 37
water-soluble vitamins 34

weight loss
  myths 8, 12–3
  permanent see permanent weight loss
    & weight control
wind-chill factor 53

X Y Z

yo-yo dieting 7, 8
yogurt 43, 49

Bibliography

Exercise Physiology; Energy, Nutrition and Human Performance, 4th Edition, McArdle, Katch and Katch, Williams & Wilkins, 1996

Manual of Nutrition, 10th Edition, MAFF, 1995

Gray's Anatomy, 37th Edition, Churchill Livingstone, 1993

Töjning av Muskler, I and II, Evjenth and Hamberg, Alfta Rehab Förlag, 1980

Useful addresses

Chin-up bars:

Polar Electro Inc, 99 Seaview Blvd, Port Washington, NY 11050.
http://www.polar.fi/

Tunturi, Tunturioyörä Oy, SF 20760, Piispanristi, Finland.
Tel: +358 21 603 111   Fax: 358 21 603 323

Cycle stands:

Cycle-Ops Products, 71 West 11th Street, New York, NY 10011.
Tel: 212 924 6724

Tacx Cycletrack, Rijksstraatweg 52, 2241 BW Wassenaar, Netherlands.
Tel: 31(0)70 511 9259   Fax: 31(0)70 511 6411

Heart-rate monitors:

Polar, Leisure Systems International Ltd.
Tel: 01926 811 611   E-mail: lsisales@lsi.co.uk
Internet: http://www.polar.fi/sampola/

Acknowledgments

Authors' Acknowledgments

I should like to record my gratitude to Torje Eike for advice on the text and constant support, and to Dr. Paul Pacy for his generous advice. Torje Eike would like to thank Prof. Patrick Salter of Queen Margaret's College, Edinburgh for instilling in him a lifelong interest in anatomy and physiology, and David West for his friendship and professional support over the last decade. We would also like to thank Monica Chakraverty and Robert Ford of Dorling Kindersley for unfailing good humor and valuable advice.

Publisher's Acknowledgements

Dorling Kindersley would like to thank:
Sue Bosanko, Lorna Damms, Nicola Graimes, Nasim Mawji, Jill Scott, and Sue Sian. Thanks also to John Woodcock for his illustration work. The following pages feature food photography by Clive Streeter: 44, 46, 48.